HAVE YOU EVER?
A new approach to those situations that "torment" your life.

SUSANA YOSHIYAMA MIYAGUSUKU

Copyright © 2020 Susana Yoshiyama Miyagusuku

All rights reserved.

To you,

who are looking for answers.

ACKNOWLEDGEMENT

I thank God and my beloved Virgin Mary for guiding and for being with me every day.
My loving parents, Mario and Sue, for their love, their teachings, and their example.
My brothers, Mario and Kike, for their support, motivation and joy.
My patients and clients, whom I always learn from and who allowed me to share their stories.
Francisco Navarro Lara for his advice, teaching and motivation.
Yrma Meneses Pardo-Figueroa for helping me with the design and beautiful graphics of the book.
Cristina Taira for the diagram design and her wise suggestions.
Bettina Villena for her joy and professionalism with the author's pictures.
Fátima Castro, Norma Lean and Nicol Olavide for their love, happiness, motivation and suggestions.
My dear friend Akira Toyama Nakahodo, for his great contribution in the microvideos of this book (not included in this book).
My great friend Rosa Sabanés, for lending her beautiful voice for the audiobook (not included in this book).
Carlos Ramírez Pantoja, for the production of the audiobooks.
My special thanks to Itala Ruth Terrones Pérez, for translating this book into English and use her lovely voice in the English audiobook.
I want to thank my dear family, friends and all those who helped me in some way to make sure this book reaches you.
Yupi, for her company, warmth and playfulness that made me laugh throughout the process of writing this book.

Thank you very much!

ABOUT THE AUTHOR

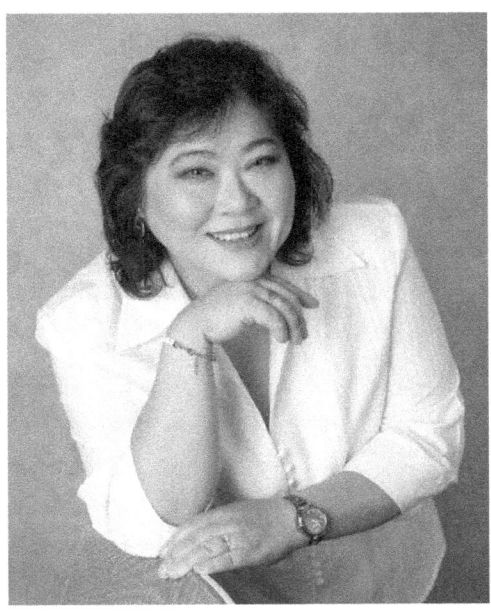

Susana Yoshiyama Miyagusuku was born in Lima, Peru, in 1972. She works a Physician-Psychiatrist, Cognitive-Behavioral Psychotherapist, international Life Coach, Executive Coach, Organizational Executive Coach, outdoor team Coach and Neuro-Linguistic Programming (NLP) practitioner. She is also a personal development expert. Susana offers private sessions, conferences, training and workshops to groups, companies and institutions in various countries. Her first book "Pintando Poesía" (Painting Poetry) was published in 1988, with remarkable success in sales. Her second book is: *"¿Te ha pasado que...?"* (Have you ever...?) This new approach to those situations that "torment" your life is the result of years of her experience as a psychiatrist, psychotherapist and coach helping thousands of people overcome "difficult" situations and reach their goals. Susana's books show great versatility. Readers are captivated by her pleasant, simple, yet deep and straightforward language.

LINKS AND E-MAIL ADDRESS

Facebook https://www.facebook.com/doctorayoshiyama

Instagram https://www.instagram.com/susanayoshiyama/

E-mail suyoshiyama@yahoo.com

TABLE OF CONTENTS

INTRODUCTION 13

CHAPTER 1 19

    What happens to you is somebody else's fault (your parents, ... 19
    your partner, your ex, your friends, your boss, etc.). 19
    Is what happens to you somebody else's fault? 19
    And why blame others for what happens to you? 22
    Do you know in what situations you usually blame others for what happens to you? 24
    What concrete actions can you take to change and accept responsibility? 25
    How do childhood experiences affect you? 26
    How did your parents shape your beliefs? 27
    What does updating data mean? 27
    Is it time to get a hold of your life? 28
    How do you reinvent yourself? 29

CHAPTER 2 33

    You do what others expect from you. 33
    Do you want to do one thing and end up doing another because what you want is not what others expect from you? 33
    Why do you do what others expect from you? 33
    How to change and stop doing what others expect from you? 35
    The two-drawing exercise. 35
    You'll probably feel chaos, it's a doodle. So what do you want for your life? 37
    You don't know how to say No! 38
    You want to be accepted. Is it *bad* that to think like this? 40
    A look that makes you unique. 41
    You put yourself off, others come first. 41
    The list exercise. 42
    Why do you accept a relationship where you only get crumbs? 43
    What can I tell you about emotional dependence? 44
    Why does someone mistreat you if you treat them well? 45
    You need your partner (or so you say). 45
    Why you don't get what you give? 46
    From peer to peer. 47
    How do you decide? 48

CHAPTER 3 51

Why don't they choose you?...51
What are the reasons why they don't choose you?......................52
What to do to avoid feeling bad if they don't choose you? 52
Each one will choose according to what they "need" specifically at that moment in their life...53
How to stop feeling something for someone that isn't good for you? 54
What to do if you have to see someone every day who didn't choose you as a partner? 55

CHAPTER 4 59

You lost motivation by losing him/her. 59
What do you mean by "loss"? 59
Why do you lose motivation when you lose someone or something important to you?..60
What to do to regain your motivation and accept the 'loss'?..........61
How to deal with guilt when you lose someone and you didn't go to see them or you think you didn't do enough?............................63
How to handle loneliness? 64
How can you overcome an empty heart? 64
How to fill the emotional void?...65

CHAPTER 5 69

How do you free yourself from the past?.....................................69
Specifically, what do you want to free yourself from?...................69
How to free yourself from the past?...69
Technique to free yourself from recurring thoughts.....................73
How to overcome negative experiences? 74
What to do so that the memory of hurtful words stops hurting?....74
How to heal emotional wounds?...75
Four steps to free yourself from the past: 77

CHAPTER 6 81

It's hard for you to take action...81
What does "taking action" mean? 81
Why is it difficult for you to take action?.....................................81
How to start taking action? 81
You want to start something and you don't. 82
How to specify what you would like to do?.................................82
You worry about what may happen. 84
How do you face the fear of what could happen, but hasn't happened yet? 85

How to stop assuming? 86
How to overcome negative emotions to go after what you want? . 87
Your brain knows it, but you do the opposite... Why? 88
You doubt yourself a lot... Will you be able to do this? 89
If you don't do it, someone else will ... Right? 90
How do you motivate yourself to get up even though you physically don't want to? 90

CHAPTER 7 95

How to keep a positive attitude in difficult situations? 95
What is a positive attitude? 95
How can you stay positive when your world is "falling apart"? 95
Understand the signs life gives you... There are no coincidences. 97
How to stay calm when dealing with emotionally disturbing situations? 98
How can you feel happy in situations that throw your heart into turmoil? 104
How to keep a good attitude towards life? 105
What helps you stay positive? 108
Thoughts that help keep a good attitude. 111
You need to have everything under control. 111
Thanks? For what? 114
How to face challenges without fear? 114
What does it mean to live fully here and now? 115
How can you find what makes you happy? 117

EPILOGUE 119

HAVE YOU EVER…?

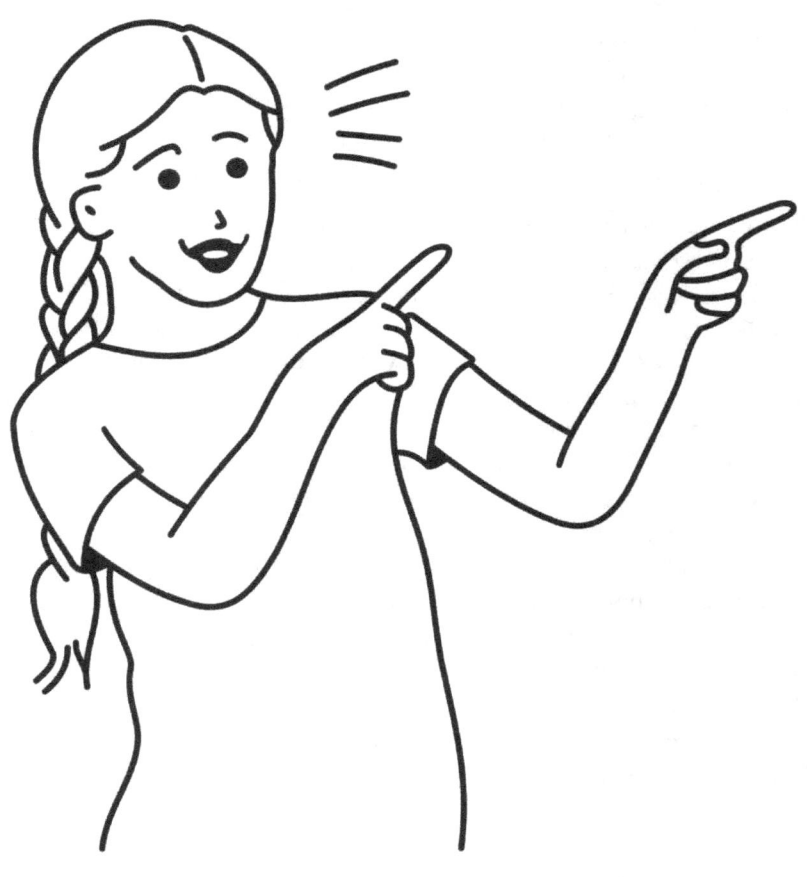

INTRODUCTION

I put this book in your hands to walk with you on this journey and this path, so that you can always count on "the other point of view" of a true friend (the one who tells you upfront because he/she loves you).

Why do you need a different point of view?

Hello! Welcome! Don't be surprised if you related to the situations I'm going to share here. It's no coincidence... I was actually waiting for you! "Have you ever...?" is a friend who shares a different approach to the different situations that "torment" your life.

A different point of view that will bring new lights to the lens you currently see the world through. It will help you focus and understand what is happening in your life, in a broader and healing way.

It will help you discover new approaches, create new strategies and solutions, to positively deal with difficult situations you're facing or have faced.

It's not what happened that really bothers you or makes you uncomfortable, but how you interpret it. If you're able to look at situations from a different angle, even if it causes you some pain, you could have the chance to break free from those negative emotions that enslave you and that prevent your life from being fuller and happier.

Those negative emotions usually block you, stop you, and keep you from moving towards your dreams (sometimes you don't even give yourself permission to dream). Having another point of view gives you the opportunity to reinterpret and update data from situations you have experienced, to be at peace with them (and with yourself) and walk in greater freedom.

Let's see...

Imagine a painting hanging on the wall: the sea, a sailboat, the sun, seagulls and palm trees. We take the painting off the wall, you look at the front of the painting and I look at the back. We are face to face and I ask you: what do you see from your side? You'll tell me: "I see a landscape, it's a picture of a sailboat in the sea, with the sun, palm trees, seagulls". I'll tell you: "from here, I see a wooden rectangle that has a crochet hook on top, but I don't see any palm tree, no sea, no sailboat or seagulls".

Whoever is between the two of us will say: "I don't see any rectangle, no palm tree, no sailboat or anything you say, I simply see an elongated rectangular edge, very thin." And the three of us will be right, each from their own point of view.

Who is telling the truth? All three! Who is wrong? None! The three of us are looking at the same object, from three different angles. If we can look at the object from different points of view, we'll have a fuller view. A single point of view is limited, biased and could be misleading.

What inspired me to write this book was seeing how my patients and clients were able to transform their lives, their thoughts, and their outlook within a few minutes, just by changing their perspective.

When I showed them another side to the situation they were going through, they drastically changed their attitude towards it. By making that *little big change*, they went from being victims of the situations to the main character of their own lives.

Seeing those changes that I've been blessed to walk them through during all these years and how it works positively to bring new points of view to the same situation, how it helps them calm down, regain confidence in themselves, rediscover who they are, how it helps them turn the page, leave the past behind, walk towards their dreams and what they want in their lives, is what inspired me to write this book.

I want to thank them and share what they taught me and the gift they gave me by trusting me (they gave me permission and the names have been changed to protect their identity). I want to share what helped them transform themselves positively, leave pain, anxiety and sadness behind and allowed them to enjoy a healthier, happier, more peaceful and fuller life. Listening to them has allowed me to create methods and strategies to help them in the best way possible throughout these years.

This book is your friend on this journey. Remember you're not alone through the difficult situations that "torment you". Remember there may be different answers than those you have already given yourself. By changing the angle of the same the situation, you can have other points of view that will help you envision new solutions, new ways of facing and dealing with the situation in a healthier, more liberated and happier way.

This book is a friend who won't judge or criticize you. It's only going to show you another point of view, perhaps different from the one you have been looking at the situation from. You may ask yourself: "And why would I need a different point of view?"

What happens is that when you see the situation from another angle, you see things that you didn't see before. More information about the situation will help you understand things better. I wish with all my heart that you can look at the situation or situations you're going through from a different angle, and that this book can help you positively change your life to a happier and fuller one.

A true and enlightening story.

When I was working in a psychiatric hospital, one day a nurse told me, "Doctor, we're about to admit a patient who burned her mom with boiling water. She threw boiling water on her mom's left side" (that was the nurse's point view, based on the information she had).

When I interviewed the patient, after mutual introduction, I asked her: "Pamela, tell me, what happened?" She told me: "Doctor, a witch was possessing my mom, just on her left side, nothing else. I poured boiling water on my mom to save her from that evil spirit, from that witch who was possessing her".

There is a popular belief that throwing boiling water at these "evil spirits" scares them away and they leave the place or the person they are "possessing or bothering".

Pamela had been diagnosed with paranoid schizophrenia and, in a visual hallucination, she had seen the spirit of a witch entering her mom's body as. By throwing boiling water at her mom, she hoped to "save" her from this "evil" spirit. Without knowing this part of Pamela's story, we could have thought that she wanted to hurt her mom... Did your view of the situation change or not when you learned of Pamela's motivation when she threw boiling water at her mom? Did she want to hurt or save her from that spirit she was seeing because of her mental illness? Things change when we realize that reality is not necessarily what we think, that when we have more information we can get a little closer to what really happened and see more clearly.

What are you going to learn?

You will learn that you are the main character of your own life, that from now on it's you who has to make the decisions in your own life. That your past, the things that have happened to you, the pains that you may have carried up to this moment, the resentment, the secrets you've kept locked away must be left behind.

You will learn that it's time to move on from all those painful and sad moments. It's time to get rid of that old suitcase you have been carrying year after year and that you keep dragging along. It's time to free yourself and leave those situations that "torment you" in the rear-view mirror.

You will learn that if you want and if you decide to do so, you can change the current situation in your life. Are you up for it?

Susana Yoshiyama Miyagusuku.

1 WHAT HAPPENS TO YOU IS SOMEBODY ELSE'S FAULT
(your parents, your partner, your ex, your friends, your boss, etc.)

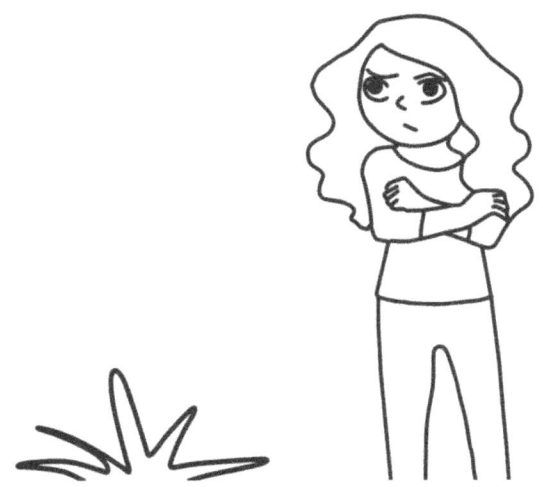

HAVE YOU EVER...?

CHAPTER 1
What happens to you is somebody else's fault (your parents, your partner, your ex, your friends, your boss, etc.).

By "others" I mean people who may have had or still have an influence in your life, in your decision-making, for example your parents, your teachers, your partner, your ex, your friends, your boss. Those people you have given permission to or have opened the door to have the power to influence you and your decisions. People who at some point in your life you decided to learn from or imitate.

Is what happens to you somebody else's fault?
We try to justify or "self-justify" many of the situations we live in by saying "I'm like this because my parents taught me", "because I saw it at home", "because that's how I experienced it", "because my teacher said it was the right thing to do", "I decided this because so and so told me", "because my friend advised me to", "I did it that way because everyone did it that way".

We consider all these kinds of situations that we live in, and that sometimes we dislike, to be the fault of our parents or of those figures who have influenced our lives. Twenty-five-year-old Felipe says "I don't have money because my dad doesn't have a job" or "I don't have a profession because my dad couldn't pay for my studies". It's true, probably his father didn't have the money to pay for his studies and did what he could, in addition to making an effort so that Felipe always had food and clothing during his childhood and teenage years.

From the moment he comes of age, Felipe can start generating income by himself. He has two arms, two legs, a brain to look for work or see how he can make money by doing something creative.

If, at twenty-five, Felipe says that he doesn't buy a chocolate bar because his father or mother doesn't give him money, what do you think of this? Is what Felipe says fair? A person of legal age can take care of himself, it's not his father's or mother's responsibility to continue feeding him until he is fifty years old.

From the moment you become an adult, you have the ability to be the one who takes responsibility for your well-being and your progress in life.

You could say "I hit my wife because I saw my father hit my mother". You may have seen that harsh, painful and unfair situation in which mom or dad beat each other, and it's true, it's not a healthy relationship, but as an adult now, you have the ability to decide whether to continue with what you saw at home or you decide to change it, that is, to do things differently, without following that example, like a sheep following the herd.

The fact that you behave in a certain way is not justified because "Blanca" told you, because she asked you to. "I got drunk at the party because my friends were forcing me to drink". Did they put a gun on your head and forced you to drink? Did they say you had to get drunk?

You must take responsibility for your decisions. Anyone can suggest "do this or do that", but any decision you make, any suggestion they give you, must go through your own filter and ask yourself, "is this good for me or not?" "Do I or do I not?"

If it seems appropriate to do what they are suggesting, you decide, "I'll do this because I've already thought it through, and I realize I should do it" and you do it. So if you do it, it's not because "someone" told you. You do it because you've already assessed the situation and decided that what they suggested was positive or appropriate for you.

Therefore, if you do it, it's your responsibility, not of the one who suggested it. If you decide not to do what Blanca suggested, great. The situation passed through your filter, you analyzed it, you decided, "what Blanca is suggesting doesn't suit me. So I decide not to do it". So, if you don't do it, it's not because you're against Blanca, but because what she told you passed through your filter, you analyzed it and decided that it wasn't convenient for you or you didn't want to do it, period. That means you're taking responsibility for your own decisions.

You decide your actions and assume their positive or negative consequences. You take responsibility (and that's what it means to grow up!). We often believe that we don't have the power to change certain situations in our lives, and we feel like we're the victims of other people or the situation.

If I'm at a job and my boss tells me to stay until 8:00 p.m. (although my shift ends at 5 p.m.), I have to stay, if not, he fires me and, even if I'm upset, I stay and say to myself, "Well, I'm going to stay because if they fire me, then I won't find another job".

I come home upset about having stayed at work late, I fight with my wife and I think, "All my problems are because of my boss". Is this true? Of course not.

Many will say, "Well, it's difficult to find work these days and you just have to put up with it". It's always been a bit hard to find a job, but it's not impossible to find it or create a new one.

It's up to you to accept the conditions or not. If you quit, you have to know that you're capable of getting a new job or of reinventing yourself and become an entrepreneur. Any job is worthy if it's done with honesty.

There are people who lost their jobs or who simply didn't want to accept unfair conditions from their bosses and decided to resign. Then, in order to keep an economic income they diversified: some began taxi driving, others knew how to knit and began to make scarves, sweaters, others knew how to make handcrafts and began to sell them, others realized that they were good in the kitchen and began to sell menus or food delivery at request.

As you can see, there are many ways to reinvent yourself. You can't say "I don't have the solution" or "I have to stay because I have no other way out".

Remember: it's not the only option. If the job you have now didn't exist, what else would you do? What would you do? I can assure you that you would be working on something anyway.

Life is not just one path. There are multiple paths leading you to your goals, to your desired results. You can reach them through different roads, through different routes, with different means. Let's say you want to go from your house to a nearby town, you can go walking, by bicycle, by car, by motorcycle, you can go by boat, by balloon, go straight ahead, going around curves, to the right, to the left, diagonally, zigzag; You can go forward, backward, turn around and go forward again.

You can also choose different people along the way, people who cheer you on and tell you keep going! One more step! Yes, you can! Or people who all day tell you, "You're useless, you don't do things well, you're late, you're not good at that". There are also people who won't tell you anything. They'll be completely indifferent to what you do.

These will be conditions that you can often decide on and sometimes not. In those where you can decide, TAKE responsibility, and in those where you cannot, you will decide how to *ecologically* manage the situation (well-being for you, those around you and the environment). If, for example, someone doesn't speak to you (and not for being introvert), perfect. You focus on your thing, you just greet and behave politely with that person.

If there is a negative person walking by your side, you decide how long you're going to stay with them or if you will talk to them the minimum necessary to get your work done, period.

All those decisions are yours. You decide what you want for your life, how and when you want it and in what different ways you can do it.

Remember there is not just one way to get things done. There are many ways to get the results you want, and you have the right to give yourself the opportunity to try these new and different ways – they may be healthier, happier or more peaceful for you.

And why blame others for what happens to you?

Most of the time you do it because you simply believe that it's really other people's fault or because you believe that you were not taught well. Perhaps because it's easier to blame others than to accept responsibility and get out of your comfort zone (a situation that is familiar to you, that you already know and know how to handle, whether you like it or not).

We are nobody to judge. Your parents, your teachers, your friends, like any other human being, have limitations and they can make mistakes. They may have learned behaviors that perhaps were not the most appropriate one, but that's what they were taught. So, we first need to understand is that, based on what they are or who they have been, even with their own limitations (the ones you know and the ones you don't), they tried to give you the best.

They tried to make you the best person they could with what they were given. We don't know exactly how or what it's that they were given when as teachings, treatment or affection. But what we do know is that based on what they are and received, they have given you something. And please, it's not that they intentionally wanted to upset you, harm you, ruin your life, hurt you or raise you negatively.

Now you can see that dad and mom are human beings who also have weaknesses, flaws, just like you and me. You can see they have not only virtues, and that they gave you the best of themselves, despite everything or with everything they were and are.

Nobody ever gives what they don't have (thanks mom and dad!) Probably, unconsciously, you think or believe that what they taught or told you - with good intentions, of course - was the only and absolute truth, and you have not realized that now it's you who decides what to do with your life.

When you were a child or a teenager (and perhaps even now) you believed that mom or dad were never wrong, that they were perfect beings, that they knew everything, and knew how to solve any problem "properly" - they were like your superheroes.

You also thought that the school teachers were wise. You blindly believed everything they taught, advised, or said. You believed that it was the right thing to do, and you made it the rule in your life, and never questioned them.

Your parents and your teachers obviously conveyed to you what they were taught, what they considered correct and they treated you probably as they were treated, believing that it was the only or the best way to treat you. Then that teaching was embedded in your mind, and you subconsciously do what you learned or saw as a child.

All was good while you were a child, but when the ability to realize if something is right or not is being shaped within you, if it should be done or not, if there are healthier or better ways to do things; when you start to question this, it's time to allow yourself to also go over these beliefs that your parents, your teachers or your friends gave you or taught you through their own example.

You now have the ability to choose what attitudes you want to keep in your life and what attitudes, beliefs, and behaviors you want to change because you don't like them, they don't suit you or simply because they don't match your values or who you are today. You have the ability to decide what you want in your life, how you want to live it, what attitudes you want to have, what way of thinking is the one that makes you feel better. So, you can't say, "I am like this because my mom or dad taught me that's how things were". They may have taught you what they considered to be the best. However and with all due respect, you now have the ability to think: Is this what I want for my life?

If so, perfect, continue with those teachings, stay with the ones that help you move forward, that are useful, that make you feel good, that generate positive feelings within you, well-being for you and those around you. But with those teachings, thoughts and actions that make you feel bad, that sadden or upset you, you have the right and the ability to say "I don't want that in my life", so I want and **decide to change** my way of thinking or doing this or my attitude towards this situation. You learn and create habits to be able to transform what you no longer want in your life.

The moment you realize that you're not your parents, you will realize that you have the right to have your own thoughts and feelings, that you have the ability to modify (if you wish) the way you think, how you interact, how you react in different situations. You will be able to lead your own life as yours. You can learn, work on it in therapy, see the most convenient and appropriate way for you, to learn and apply the behaviors and thoughts of the person you want to be in your life.

When you take responsibility for your life, you stop blaming or giving others credit for what you're today. It's time to update the data and now become your own superhero.

Do you know in what situations you usually blame others for what happens to you?

It's usually in situations that don't turn out the way you wanted-those situations that frustrate you (Grrrrrrr!)

Imagine you're in a relationship and suddenly he/she breaks up with you. He/she tells you that he/she no longer loves you and wants to leave the relationship. So go under the covers in your bed, go in fetal position, you don't want to go out, you don't want to bathe, you don't want to have a social life, you lock yourself in your world and say "my life is a mess because of my ex", "I don't go to work or study".

Let's see... Is your ex forcing you not to get out of bed, not to bathe? Or is it you who decided not to do it because you feel sad, with no energy or desire for anything? Is anyone forcing you to stay like this?

Of course ending a relationship is a painful situation. You can feel sad, you want to cry, you don't want to do things, but you decide if you surrender to that lack of desire to do anything or if despite the pain or even with it, you start (even if it's hard) to get up and out of bed, bathe, go out with friends. It's all up to you.

What concrete actions can you take to change and accept responsibility?

The first thing is to realize how you have been living and acting until today. Did you assess the decisions you have been making? Did you wonder: Do I want this or not? Does it suit me or not? Or were you almost automatically doing what you saw other people do (parents, teachers, friends)? Did you just mimic these attitudes or did you think before acting? It's the first thing you have to analyze.

Once you have detected what actions you want to modify, ask if it's what you want for your life, if you feel better or worse with them, if it's convenient for you to maintain those attitudes or not. If you say "I want to keep this attitude in my life despite everything", then stay with it. If you say "I don't want to continue with this attitude, I want to change it", then think what different behavior, what different attitude you want to have, and start practising, one step at a time, one day at a time - slowly but surely.

If out of ten times, nine are the old habits and one is the new behavior that you want to have. Congratulations! That is already a step forward! Be patient and consistent with yourself. Keep moving forward. Next time, the old attitudes will be seven times out of ten and three will be the new ones. That way, little by little, you will make progress until you reach a point where the new desired behavior will automatically emerge.

At the beginning, you will need to be very aware of how you're doing things in those specific situations (like someone who watches carefully). At first it is a bit hard, but it's easy to implement, and you can do it little by little. I'm not asking you to change your attitudes overnight. It's enough that one attitude out of then is modified, and you'll keep moving forward little by little. That is one of the ways how you change and take responsibility for your new decisions. The next thing: you start listening to your language because the person who blames others for what happens to them uses a lot of what I call "the goat language" (*mee mee*, like the sound the goats make), the victim's language.

The victim says "They made *me* suffer", "they made *me* cry", "they rejected *me*", "I ... I ..." It's important to modify this "goat language" for the language of the protagonist or survivor, meaning, to start with "*I*". For example "*I* felt sad when that happened", "*I* take responsibility for this emotion that *I* am feeling"; It's not "they made me feel sad". "*I* was angry when this happened" rather than "they made *me* angry".

If you use the "goat language", you give all your power to the other person. So, since the other person is (apparently) "guilty" of what happens to you, he/she is also the only one who could save you or get you out of that situation. On the other hand, if you use the "*I*' language", with the "*I*" ahead, as in "*I* feel sad because José did not come to see me", what you do when you speak this way is to assume responsibility for your emotions, for your attitudes.

Therefore, if you're responsible for your feelings, you'll also be responsible and capable of modifying or changing what you feel, if you wish, because it's you who decides, not anyone else. The power is within you.

How do childhood experiences affect you?

During childhood, you're like a sponge: you absorb everything that happens to you. What you see, what you feel, the way they treat you, how they talk to you, what they tell you, what they teach you, everything is recorded. In most cases, how you learn to look at the world starts at home: from the example you see in your own home, and then what you see later in teachers, classmates, friends. The foundations of the lenses you will use to start looking at the world are shaped there (and you'll believe that the world looks "only" that way).

You register what happened to you in childhood with the amazing intensity of children and their delicate vulnerability. However, those things are not necessarily going to determine your present or your future - they can be modified. But how? By changing beliefs and your outlook on the current situation (in your adolescence or adulthood). The impact would be different if the same situation happens to a child or an adult.

Have you ever been hit by a wave? Imagine you're five and you're on the beach really enjoying the warm water of the sea, playing with your sand buckets, and suddenly a "huge" (for you, at that age) wave comes and it knocks you over, you swallow salt water, and your face gets sand all over while you spin around underwater. After that experience, you most likely won't want to go back into the sea for a long time. Suppose you're now twenty years old and when you go to the beach you only stay on the sand or walk along the shore. You're still afraid of the sea (you politely say, "I don't go in because I have respect for the sea").

In order to give yourself the opportunity to enjoy the sea again, it's important that you update data that you realize that now you're a strong, big, twenty-year-old person, with greater stability, who will hardly be rolled over by a wave like a five-year-old child. You will say then: "When I was five years old, I did not have the strength or the stability that I have now at twenty years of age" so the circumstances and the ways have changed, so the results will be different.

How did your parents shape your beliefs?

In your childhood your parents were your first source of beliefs because they were the ones who told you "don't get on that chair, you can fall", "men never cry", "good girls are obedient", and so on. Many of the beliefs that you've kept until today have to do with those words your parents taught you in childhood.

Your first years of life are the most important stage to register and learn how you'll face the world. In childhood, you're shaping the first points of view that you'll use throughout life. Little by little, those beliefs that you're learning at home are embedded in your brain, by constant repetition.

When something is repeated thirty to three hundred times, it's recorded at the subconscious level and the behavior happens almost automatically. However, the good news is that what was recorded at a subconscious level can be replaced by new beliefs that can be installed in our mind, by personal choice.

What does updating data mean?

Your mind "recorded" situations that had an emotional impact on you at a certain age and although time passed, you still feel or remember them as if you were at the age when they happened to you.

It may also be that you feel as if the circumstances were the same as those present on that occasion (even if years had passed).

Updating data means looking at the same past situation but with your current age, at the present time, with the new personal resources that you have now. For example, your father scolded you when you were seven, the intensity of the scolding and its pain is very intense because you were a seven-year-old child and it impacted you very hard.

Suppose that you're now twenty years old, and your father scolds you again with the same intensity as when you were seven years old, the impact will be much less because you're now an adult. When your dad would scold you when you were seven, you would run away crying. But now that you're twenty, if your dad scolds you, you listen, if you have to respond, you'll do it politely and then leave without drama. That's how you update your data.

Have you ever been in a situation that when people ask you what your personality is like, you listed characteristics you thought of at some point in your life (usually during puberty or adolescence): "How am I? I'm shy, I'm smart, I don't know how to speak in public", etc.

Now, at thirty, they ask you again: "What are you like?" And you keep repeating the same words and concepts. However, I assure you that many things have happened in your life during these years, various experiences and much changed in you. Maybe you're no longer the introverted girl you were (because you went through high school or college, you had to learn how to speak in public, interact and give a presentation in class).

You're now a talkative, friendly girl who can easily speak in public. Then you have to update data, stop repeating what you say about yourself as if you were repeating a script (just because you thought about it at some point in your life).

You would have to say now: "Before, when I was twelve years old, I was shy, intelligent and did not dare to speak in public. Now in my 30s, after updating data, I am a friend, I interact well with people, I am intelligent and I speak easily in public". This way, you'll be updating data in the different areas of your life.

Is it time to get a hold of your life?

With what you've read so far, you realize that much of what happens to you (or everything) has to do with taking responsibility. You have to realize that others are not responsible for what happens to you or your decisions. The only person who owns your decisions and is responsible for them is you. Bingo!

The time has come to be responsible for yourself, to own your own decisions and therefore take responsibility for your life and for what you decide for yourself in **your life**.

How do you reinvent yourself?

One of the most beautiful ways to reinvent yourself is to first realize how lucky you are to have, in your hands, the ability and the beautiful responsibility to decide how you want to be, how you want to live, face, flow and enjoy your life from now on.

You're the one who decides what goal and dreams you want to achieve. By reinventing yourself, it's you who will enhance those qualities you want to develop within. You'll learn new skills to achieve your most beautiful dreams or goals.

Reinventing yourself is assuming, with joy and hope, the beautiful responsibility of being the one who will create and recreate the human being that you want to be, with the qualities and abilities you want to have.

Nobody is born with all the qualities and all the flaws at once, nobody is 100% qualities or 100% flaws. To be complete human beings, all of us have, on the one hand, our qualities and on the other our flaws.

Reinventing yourself has to do with enhancing the qualities you already have. It has to do with learning those new skills you want to acquire. It has to do with polishing or dismissing those attitudes that you don't like about yourself (suddenly those "ugly" things that you tell yourself secretly, the "unfair" way you treat yourself or others), attitudes, thoughts that you decide to change for your own good. You have the power to decide how you want to live. Slowly (with joy and hope), start strengthening those qualities, attitudes and beliefs that will help you become the person you want to be and that will become the stepping stool to your most beautiful dreams.

Congratulations!

HAVE YOU EVER...?

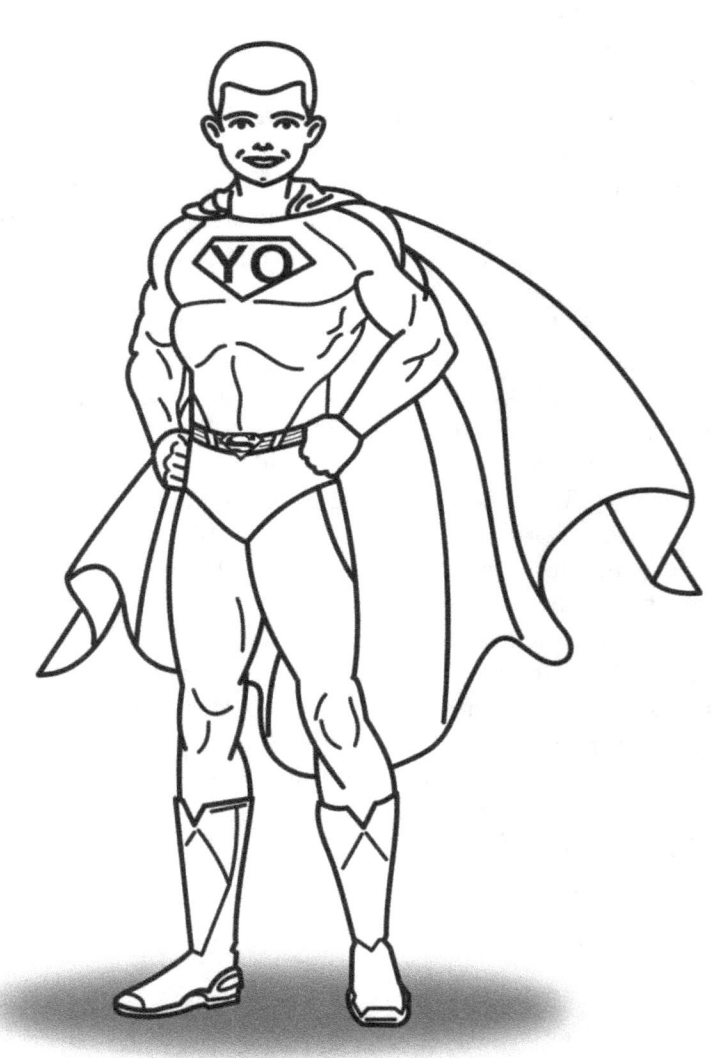

2 YOU DO WHAT OTHERS EXPECT FROM YOU

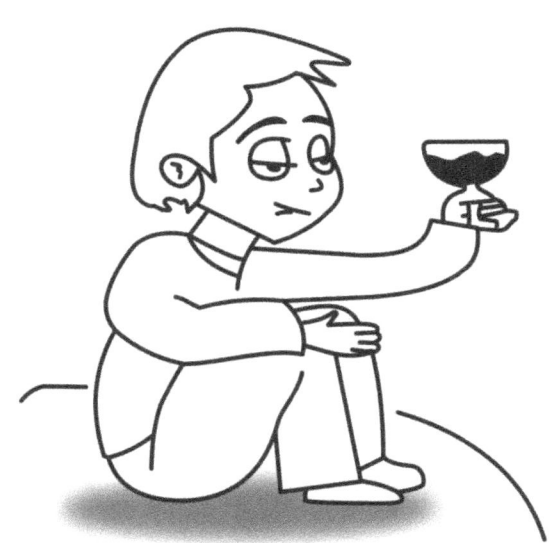

HAVE YOU EVER…?

CHAPTER 2

You do what others expect from you.

Do you want to do one thing and end up doing another because what you want is not what others expect from you?

"I would like to be a painter, study art, but everyone in my family wants me to be a lawyer or a business administrator (or any other profession)". So, to please your family, you go and study law, not because it's your vocation, but because it's what they expect from you. And you want your parents, siblings and those who know you to feel proud of you. You want to feel accepted by them.

"I like to dress casually, with a T-shirt, blue jeans. But when I go out to dinner with my friends, they want me to wear a formal shirt and pants, so I totally change the way I dress when I go out to dinner with them because it's what they expect of me (even if I don't feel comfortable, I do what is necessary to feel accepted by them)".

"My name is Ramiro and I like to knit, sew and do crafts. My family tells me that these activities are for women, to stop doing them and to start playing soccer (although I'm not interested) and to stop my passion for crafts".

"When I'm at a party or a meeting, my friends tell me that to show that I am part of the group I should have a few beers. But I don't like to drink alcohol, I prefer plain water, but I have to have a few beers to be accepted in this group".

You actually don't have to drink. I know you feel peer pressure and that's probably why you end up drinking (it's what they expect of me - you might say). You're still changing what you wanted to do by wanting to feel accepted by the group, by being part of it, by "belonging".

Why do you do what others expect from you?
Reasons to do what others expect from you:

- Lack of self-confidence, of the ability to do something for yourself and to do it well.
- Fear of making a mistake, of making the wrong choice.
- You want to feel accepted by them.
- It's easier to do what others tell you and not take responsibility for your decisions and their consequences. For example: It's more comfortable for someone to tell you what to do and for you to do it to the letter. If you fail, you'll say, "Ah ... I did it because Rodrigo told me to do it like that," so it's Rodrigo's "fault" that you didn't do things properly. And if it goes well, great, you just accept that things went well.

You seek acceptance, to be on the same page as others, integrate. You want to feel that you belong to a group, a family, an institution and that others trust you. It's scary to be original because you fear of criticism, not being loved, not being chosen if you don't behave as is expected of you.

Sometimes, when you want to feel loved by someone, you change the way you are, you excessively try to please the other person, even when your desires, concerns and habits are different from the other person's expectations. So let me ask you: What price are you paying to be accepted and loved by someone else?

Miguel has extraordinary human qualities: He is friendly, inclusive, likes to interact with all kinds of people, belongs to a high socioeconomic class, enjoys sharing in meetings with his workers, talking with them and treating them as equals (not as a boss). However, his wife strongly disagrees with him and tells him that she should not spend time with his company's employees, that he should not share a coffee or a few beers with them because "they are not of his socioeconomic class" and she refuses to be with him in these get-togethers.

Every time Miguel spends time with his company workers, a war breaks out at home: His wife, Marcela, is very upset by these get-togethers. Regardless of whether or not you agree with Marcela's reaction, you should know and understand that she was raised that way, with certain beliefs (whether rational or irrational).

I'm not making any kind of judgment, nor am I siding with anyone. I am simply giving an example. Miguel, in order to maintain peace in his marriage, stopped holding social gatherings with his employees.

Months passed, and Miguel felt sad, moody, he really enjoyed spending time with all his workers, and he stopped doing it "to keep the peace" with his wife at home.

He got to the point where one day he said, "I can't take it anymore, I like sharing with my workers. To please my wife or to be at peace with her, should I just stop doing what I enjoy? I'm not hurting anyone". When Miguel started to participate in the get-togethers with his workers again, he smiled again, he felt authentic again and said, "I'm not going to lose my authenticity to please my wife. This is me and I like sharing with my workers. If she doesn't like the people I spend time with, then unfortunately she will have to learn to respect my friends or my decisions. If she agrees, fine, and if she doesn't, it will be a reason to see if we are meant to share our lives together or not".

How to change and stop doing what others expect from you?
Remember, you have the right to choose the lifestyle you want. The people who love you the most can make suggestions. They can tell you "do this or do that" with the best intention, with the best intention. However, life is yours and only you have the right to decide on it.

Original people are much more attractive and happier than those who are simply a "copy" or those who do what other people expect them to do.

The two-drawing exercise.
Let's do an exercise:
• Get two equal size blank sheets, and a box of color pencils (or various colors).
• On one of the blank sheets, make a free drawing, whatever you want and use any colors you want. Take the time you need and draw what you want. I only ask that you do the drawing now, before moving on to the next point.
• Done? If you haven't, please do it right now. In order for this exercise to have the desired effect or impact, you need to make a free drawing, whatever you want, using the colors you want.
• Now take the other blank sheet, choose a color pencil and divide it into three equal parts, with lines.
• Choose another pencil color and draw lots of circles of different sizes, all over the sheet, but not touching the lines dividing the sheet.
• Now you're going to make triangles (again please choose another pencil color), each triangle will be made up of three circles (of which you have already drawn). Join the circles from their centers, to form

each triangle. You can't use the same circles that you already used to make other triangles. Build as many triangles as you can.

• Choose another color pencil, and draw "hashtags" of different sizes all over the page.

• Take another color pencil and start making "rays" of different sizes and different directions. Count to twenty while you draw and stop.

• Finally, choose a dark color and scribble all over the page, like a five-year-old; do your worst scribble all over the page, continue until everything is well scribbled, count to thirty and stop.

Now look at both of your drawings, on the same type of sheets and with the same pencils. Now I ask you:

☐ What do you see when you look at both drawings?

☐ Which of the two pictures gives you more peace?

☐ Which of the two makes the most sense to you?

☐ Which of the two drawings was easier for you to make?

☐ Which drawing most clearly conveys the message that you wanted to give?

Do you have the answer? Good. Note that both drawings are made by the same person, on the same type of sheets and with the same color pencils. However, the results are completely different.

The first drawing you made is clean, has a defined shape. This probably expresses what you wanted to convey. Perhaps when you look at that drawing, it conveys greater peace. The other drawing that was also made by you, on the same type of sheet, with the same color pencils, what do you feel when you look at it?

You'll probably feel chaos, it's a doodle. So what do you want for your life?
In the first drawing, you made your own decisions, chose the colors and drew what came to your mind or what was born from your heart. It's something yours, original, something of your own.

Now look at the result of the other drawing (the second one). Apparently, I let you choose the colors, but, with the "best" intention, I was telling you what you had to draw, how long to do it, when you had to stop and change. I may have directed you with the best intention, but what was the result?

Have you ever been in this situation? You start doing something and suddenly someone tells you: "No, not that way, it's better this way". So, do you stop what you were doing to do something else and you keep changing and changing? In the end, the result of your life is like that drawing, a doodle ... How do you feel living your life like this? ... Like a "doodle".

That is the importance of assuming your own life, that you realize how important it's that you trust yourself. When you allow yourself to manifest what is within you, I guarantee you: the result will be beautiful, it will make sense, it will radiate peace, tranquility, well-being. You will manifest your own true self.

"I'm afraid of being wrong" you say. Everything that comes from you spontaneously is valid, original, valuable because it comes from you, from someone original, from someone with totally different experiences from other people.

Therefore, you're an original being and what you share, what you believe, what you give, will be totally original and valid. No one will have the right to say "it's good or it's bad", no one can judge you (if they do, it's their problem, not yours).

You should be proud to share your originality, not the things you copy ("I say this because I heard my friend say it the other day").

I ask you in all honesty, who are the people you're most attracted to? Those who follow others like little sheep or those who say what they think, who express their emotions and are original (that is, who show themselves as they truly are)? What kind of people are you most attracted to?

Original people are actually more attractive because there are plenty of copies and you don't have to be one of the bunch. If you're a unique, special creation, and no one in the world is the same as you, you have the opportunity to share that original gift of being you. You don't have to copy anyone. Trust that you've come with a unique gift into this world, and that it's priceless if you allow yourself and dare to share your gift with those around you and with the world.

You don't know how to say No!

Difficulty saying "no" is more a lack of assertiveness (in this case being "passive") than being "nice". What do I mean by "lack of assertiveness?" Being assertive is enforcing your rights, but respecting the rights of others.

It's someone capable of saying yes when he/she wants to say yes and saying no when he/she wants to say no - always with respect to himself/herself and others.

On the one hand, there is the passive person, the one who allows them to step on his/her rights, who doesn't know how to say no, who always says yes (even if they don't want to or don't agree). Then, we also have the aggressive person, who doesn't respect anyone's rights, and just enforces his/her own.

Let's look at the passive, assertive, and aggressive person in the following simple examples:

1. - It's very cold, Jose has a coat on, because he is very cold, and Pedro asks him to lend him his coat.

- The **passive** person: Jose takes off his coat and gives it to Pedro immediately.
- The **assertive** person: Jose tells Pedro that he would love to lend him his jacket, but that he will not do so because he feels very cold.
- The **aggressive** person: Jose tells Pedro not to bother him, to figure it out, and to go buy his own jacket wherever the hell he can.

2. - Just five minutes before leaving work, Omar, Liliana's boss, tells her that she has to submit a report at 8:00 a.m. The next day, Liliana agrees and stays working late into the night at the office and even takes the remaining work home to finish it.

The next day she leaves without breakfast and arrives all baggy-eyed at the office, but she manages to submit the report to her boss, as he had requested. In this case, we're not referring to a responsible worker. Here Liliana didn't know how to be an assertive person.

She could've assertively said to her boss, "Look, Omar, I'll be happy to give you the report, but it won't be ready early tomorrow. I'm leaving the office in five minutes. I'll do it first thing tomorrow morning and as soon as I finish it I'll give it to you".

Many people are afraid to say no because they think that by giving a different opinion or denying the request will make them look "problematic" or "bad"; but it's not like that. You have the right to refuse to do what you don't want to do, you have the right to have a different opinion, to take care of yourself and take care of what is important to you.

3. - Claudia is a doctor, she has not slept because she has been working from 8:00 a.m. until 8:00 p.m. She is about to go out to rest, but her colleague Marlene asks her to please stay and cover for her until 2:00 a.m. because she wasn't going to be able to come to the hospital. Then, instead of saying "I'm sorry, I can't stay, I'm exhausted, I want to go home and rest", she says "Sure, don't worry, I'll stay".

The truth is that Claudia doesn't want to stay to cover her colleague's shift, but she thinks if she says no to Marlene, she will be annoyed or upset. Or, if she was her boss, she thinks she could fire her from her job.

When anyone says no to someone's request, the other person will feel uncomfortable (it's normal, right?). But if the person is mature, they will soon understand and *voila*. If they're not mature and get upset, it will be their problem, not yours.

4. - Let your imagination fly for a moment, let go... OK? Imagine that you're Roberto and you're 38 years old. Now imagine that you, Roberto, are a five-year-old boy and this Roberto is asked to sweep and clean the whole house. He has already done his work and then Eduardo comes and asks him now to clean all the windows for him and the bathrooms as well because he is tired and doesn't want to clean them.

You, Roberto, the adult, has to take care of Roberto, the child. Eduardo, the adult, has to take responsibility for the things that Eduardo, the child, has to do.

If you don't take care of Roberto, the child, no one will be responsible for taking care of him. No one will come to tell you "How hard you have worked, you deserve a star on your forehead!" You understand?

If Roberto, the child, gets sick, Roberto, the adult, will have to take care of him. Roberto, the adult, is responsible for taking care of the well-being, health and tranquility of Roberto, the child. Each one of us is responsible for taking care of his inner child. So take responsibility for yours.

5. - If there is a lunch and they tell you "there are only ten dishes, but we are eleven people, then you're going to run out of food", if you answer, "No problem, let the others eat, I won't eat. I don't matter", you're not being responsible or fair to yourself. You're feeding the rest of the children and not yours.

The Solomonic thing would be to say "We distribute the ten dishes among all", but you do not leave your inner child hungry, simply because someone asks you to.

You have the right to say no, you have the right to take care of yourself. You have to know that the other person can be uncomfortable when you say no, that it's normal. You have to know that you're not the only person who can do them favors or that you have to solve their life. If you were not there at that time, they would ask someone else for help and if they didn't find someone else, they would find a way to do it themselves.

Start taking care of your inner child, because nobody else, no matter how much they love you, is going to be able to do it (even if they wanted to). Each person is responsible for their inner child, i.e., for themselves.

You want to be accepted. Is it *bad* that to think like this?

It's natural to want to be accepted by others. However, the truth is that 50% of people will like you, and the other 50% won't. Whatever you do, positive or negative, 50% will agree with you, and the other 50% will criticize you (for whatever reason, real or not).

Everyone has the right to have a different opinion than you or me, so not everyone will agree with you, with your attitudes, with what you say or feel. But, what others say is their business, not yours.

It's important for you to accept yourself as you are. Remember that you're unique and that you have the right to your own opinions and decisions, that you can be faithful to yourself without thinking about what others will say (the famous "What will they say?") or if the rest will accept or not what you decide to be or do. As long as you're calm with yourself and with your decisions, everything will be fine.

Let yourself speak, listen to yourself and allow yourself to be you, not others' project. You're not playdough or anyone's puppet for them to do whatever they want with you. You're an original being. Allow yourself to be who you are, how you're born, how you want to be. Be aware that you don't need others' acceptance. You want to be accepted, but you don't need to be.

A look that makes you unique.

A few years ago I was driving and I stopped at a red light, I was approached by a boy, about eight years old, who was selling candy. The truth is I had no intention of buying candy, but I lowered the window, looked him in the eye and asked, "What's your name?" The boy looked up and answered: "Juan Carlos" with a big smile from ear to ear while his little eyes were shining. I asked him how old he was, he told me he was eight.

I told him that he was a beautiful little boy with a beautiful smile. His smile was a gift that made my day. This short dialogue was enough to see how his little face lit up. In that moment, I realized how important it's to stop, look people in the eye, and ask them or say something positive about them.

The "What's your name?" then became a look that made that person feel unique from others. It helped the other person feel special, unique, accepted and recognized by someone - even if only for a moment.

You put yourself off, others come first.

Please pay attention to the phrase: **"make yourself a priority"**. It's time to do it.

Until today, you may have put off too much for other people's sake, but it's time you put yourself first. That doesn't mean that you become selfish, we are not saying all should be for you and nothing for the rest. Don't confuse selfishness with self-esteem or self-care. It's time you took care of yourself.

Imagine everyone is responsible for their hungry four-year-old child. If you procrastinate and feed everyone except your child and leave him hungry, how do you think he would feel being ignored by you? What emotions would come to his heart? Sadness, anger, crying, rebellion, discouragement, probably many negative emotions.

Remember that each adult is responsible for their inner child, therefore, your responsibility lies with your inner child, others' inner children have their own adults to take care of them. You take care of yours because no other person is going to do it for you. It's important that you do things for yourself and take care of yourself.

Let's do an exercise to start making yourself a priority:

The list exercise.

You will need two papers and a pen. Ready? Let's start…

The first sheet will be titled "The things I do for the people I love" and write ten things you do for the people you love.

For example "go with them to the doctor when they're in poor health". What else do you do for the people you love? Maybe "call them and ask them how they are and spend a little time with them". What else do you do for the people you love? "I hug them, I kiss them, I prepare their breakfast, their lunch, I tell them jokes to make them smile, I buy them gifts" or "I have small gestures for them", for example, if I know they like chocolate cake, I buy it for them.

On the other blank sheet, write as a title "The things that people who love me do for me" and write ten things that people who love you do for you. For example "They visit me, they accompany me to the places I want to go, they send me loving messages, they encourage me when I feel sad".

Once you have finished both lists, read everything you do for other people and what other people do for you.

What do you realize? Yes, you're a person who gives affection and also receives affection through different actions.

What else do you realize? That both, you and other people, do positive things for each other, to show the love they have for each other. As you know, and have recognized, you have done things for people you love or care for. You already have the experience of doing these things. Therefore, those same things you do for others, you're going to start doing them for yourself now.

For example, if you prepare the best breakfast for someone you love, then you're going to buy the best bread, ham, cheese, butter, eggs, fruits, yogurt (whatever you want). You're going to prepare the best breakfast for yourself. And you're going to say to yourself: "I do this for me and for myself, because I am important to me".

You're a person who calls on the phone to ask others, "How are you?" Well, now you'll stop and ask yourself, "How am I today?" You'll listen to your answer and you'll say to yourself, "What can I do to feel happier?" You'll do the entire list you wrote, but this time you'll do the actions for yourself. As you also have the experience of having received what other people who love you do for you, those actions have served as an example and **now you're going to start doing them yourself, for yourself.**

For example, if the people who love you accompany you to the places you want to go (even if they have to get up at dawn to go with you), the next time, even if you're lazy, you will get out of bed and if you want to go to the beach you will accompany yourself, and take yourself to the beach for a walk. You understand? It's about you doing for yourself what the people who love you have already done for you. This is a practical, simple and pleasant way to start taking care of yourself with love.

Why do you accept a relationship where you only get crumbs?

You accept a relationship where you're given crumbs because when you "starve", you accept what they give you. Those who are "starving" will find that even a stale piece of bread is delicious, and they will eat it. If there is an "emotional void" in you, you'll likely try to fill it or cover it with anything similar to love. That is how you agree to receive "crumbs" in the love department.

Rebeca was in a relationship and her partner, Carlos, abused her psychologically. He would tell her that she didn't know how to dress, that she was ugly, that she was stupid and useless. He'd only approach her when he wanted to be intimate. She felt used and wondered: "Why do I accept crumbs from Carlos?" Rebeca felt a great emotional emptiness (her mother passed away when she was born and her father didn't have time to care for her because he had to work to support her). She believed that the pseudo-love that Carlos gave her would fill her emotional needs, but every time he'd approach her, she felt even emptier because she realized that she was accepting "crumbs".

You know, the affective void is not filled thanks to the presence of another person in your life or with one or many things. It is filled with your own unconditional love towards yourself.

Imagine yourself as an adult and as your inner child (Juana and Juanita, respectively). You see, Juanita is only going to be cared for by

Juana, not by someone else's adult. Therefore, you'll begin to take care of yourself, so that you can begin to love yourself. Loving yourself unconditionally will make you feel fulfilled. "But how do I go about loving myself unconditionally?" Accepting you as you are, with all your virtues and defects, as you are, without feeling ashamed of any aspects of you or trying to hide them.

Then starting to take care of yourself, just as you take care of other people, start to take care of you. Just as you accompany others to the doctor, if you have any discomfort, start taking yourself to the doctor to get better. Start to take care of yourself, to be important to yourself. Do you think a fulfilled person would accept a stale piece of bread to eat? It's very likely that that person who is not hungry and goes to a pastry shop or bakery, will look for something that they really crave and want, and won't buy a hard piece of bread.

What can I tell you about emotional dependence?

You depend on another person when you don't take care of yourself. Affective dependencies tell us that there are "emotional gaps" (hidden inside), and you falsely believe that someone else will fill that emotional void. Without realizing it, you place your partner as the sun in your life, and you become the planet that revolves around it. Your decisions and actions depend on what your partner does or doesn't do.

You change what you wanted to do to be next to your significant other. And if they are not there, you feel as if something is missing, you get anxious, you feel blocked if you're not by their side or if you did not run a decision by them. You literally put your life into someone else's hands. Remember, your emotional stability cannot be in someone else's hands because no matter how much that person loves or even with their best intentions, they could unintentionally let you fall and break you.

With unconditional love for yourself, it's you who is going to fill that emotional gap. You're going to make yourself complete and feel complete all around. By loving yourself, you'll be able to really love someone else. You'll be able to autonomously enjoy a relationship with your partner. Otherwise, we could be talking about self-deception (you think you'd "die of love" for someone, when in reality, you may just be trying to fill that emotional need).

I'll give you a clear example: It's as if you were hungry and put incense or music to satisfy your hunger. You know well that it won't solve the problem. If you want to calm your hunger, you'll have to eat something. Incense or music will distract you momentarily, but you'll still be hungry. So, if you're hungry, eat! You have to do what is necessary. If you feel that inner emptiness, it's important that you begin to love yourself and complete yourself with your own love.

Why does someone mistreat you if you treat them well?

Each person gives according to what they are and what they have. If you're a source of pure water, what are you going to offer? Obviously pure water. If the other person is a source of contaminated water, what will they offer? Contaminated water. Each one gives what they are and what they have.

What the other person does speaks of them, of what they are, of what they are made of, of the way they were raised, how they decided to lead their life. The way you react, the way you respond, talks about you, talks about who you are, and talks about what you have within.

You need your partner (or so you say).

Have you ever found it hard to differentiate between what is a need (something vital, essential to survive, such as water or air) and something that you want with all your heart (such as loving or caring about someone)?

"I need my partner". No, you don't need them, you love them. You want their presence, but not everything you want you can (or should) have whenever you want it. Sometimes it happens, sometimes it doesn't. Sometimes they're there, sometimes they aren't. No partner is essential.

We do not "need", we love. What happens when you put yourself in a position of "need?" It's like making putting yourself in a victim position. In this position, you simply reach out, as if you were asking for crumbs. A happy, calm, or emotionally balanced relationship can never occur in a victim-executioner relationship (one with power and the other without power).

Esther came to my office when she was 72 years old. She had been married to Manuel for over fifty years. He was an outstanding university professor, while she didn't have the opportunity to complete her primary studies. Esther felt inferior in front of her husband. He treated her as if she had to serve him. He spoke to her in a curt, cold way. He never asked her for her opinion about anything, and she maintained that handicapped attitude for not having completed her primary studies.

When Esther began therapy, we worked on her self-esteem, on realizing that not having completed her studies didn't make her less of a person than her husband or anyone. We saw how valuable her opinions were because she had life experience, and life teaches through experience. Not everything is learned in the classroom. Perhaps what is essential has more to do with the values we have, with the priorities in our lives, with spirituality. Esther improved her self-esteem, and gradually allowed an attitude of greater respect towards herself, of greater validation regarding the things she did, and greater security in the decisions she made.

After a few months of therapy, her husband began to look at her with respect. He asked for her opinion, he ran things by her, and he even started setting up the table to have lunch and supper together. At night, if she fell asleep before him, Manuel gave her a kiss on the forehead and covered her tenderly with the blanket (Esther told me that she noticed one day when she wasn't "so asleep"). Before, Manuel was totally indifferent to her. But the moment Esther started to value herself, she began to smile, to see her own worth, he too began to look at her "as equals", to see her as a very valuable human person. Now they're both happy and respect each other.

Why you don't get what you give?

Have you ever treated people well, have beautiful gestures for them, worry about their well-being and yet you don't receive a similar response? You can say "I don't do things expecting a response or retribution", and it's true. At the time you did it, you didn't expect any similar response. However, when time passes and you start to analyze things, you say, "I've always been willing to help them. In fact, I've treated them well and yet they never have a considerate response towards me. Rather, it's as if they never have any gestures towards me, and that hurts, it's tiring".

You don't do things because you're expecting an equal reaction, but you certainly at least expect something similar in a similar situation. From my point of view, each one is like a different bottle. A bottle? Imagine that you're a three-liter bottle, and the other person is a half-liter bottle. When you give your three liters, you can give too much to the other person. You can also give just a bit of yourself and fill that person (half-liter bottle). But maybe that half-liter bottle person gives you 100% of it, and for you it won't be enough (as if that person had done almost nothing for you).

So, it's not that the other person doesn't want to do something for you, it's that their capacity is different from yours. You're someone with a greater capacity and even if the other person gives you their 100%, it still won't be enough. That's why not everyone responds in the same way. You don't know exactly what the other person's responsiveness is. So, when you do something for someone, just do it from your heart, and forget what you did for that person because their response doesn't depend on you. It depends on the other person's responsiveness.

It will also depend on their upbringing, their values, the examples they've had in their life, their life history and background, possible traumas, etc. It may be different factors that make a person respond or react in one way or another. This has nothing to do with whether they love you or not, whether or not you're important to them. It has to do with their upbringing, their own story, their values, with how that person is and how they manifest themselves to others.

From peer to peer.

When I was eleven, I was in my room, studying for a school test. I was probably a bit nervous because my grandmother (who was Japanese) came in and in her limited Spanish, she told me "Susy, don't be afraid, the teacher is a person, a human being, just like you", and added, "The teacher is an older person, with studies, but they are people, human beings, just like you ... So, don't be afraid, because they are people, human beings, just like you".

That was one of the most important messages I've ever received in my life. Thanks to those words, to that teaching, I can talk to anyone, regardless of their social status, and I assure you that I look at the person, not at their position, race or socioeconomic status.

When I was talking with Mariela about treating people equally, even if they are authority figures, she told me that she worked very closely with a Minister of State to whom she always said "Good morning, Mr. Minister", "Mr. Minister this, Mr. Minister that".

One morning Mariela walks in the office, greets him "Mr. Minister, good morning". Then he asks her to come over and says "I want to ask you something". "Yes, Mr. Minister, tell me", Mariela replied. "Did you poop today?" He asked her. Mariela blushed and looking down she answered, "Yes". He said: "So did I, so stop calling me Mr. Minister and let's talk on a first-name basis".

This example shows that it's not about dealing with positions or socioeconomic status. It's about dealing with human beings what really counts.

How do you decide?

When it comes to deciding, no one knows for sure which decision is the right one (maybe there is no right or wrong, just one decision). Just trust your instinct, that inner wisdom, your intuition. The best decisions are not necessarily the most analyzed ones or the ones that make us happiest at the moment, but rather those that give us peace in the long run, in our minds and in our hearts.

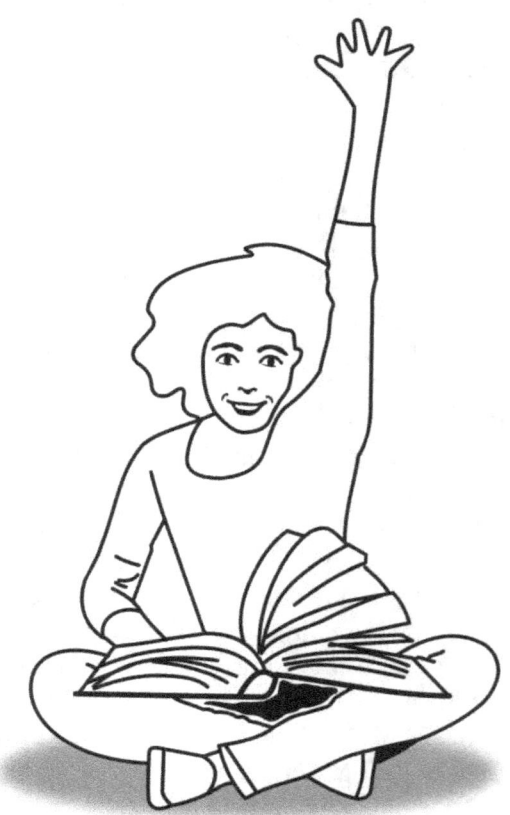

3 Why don't they choose you?

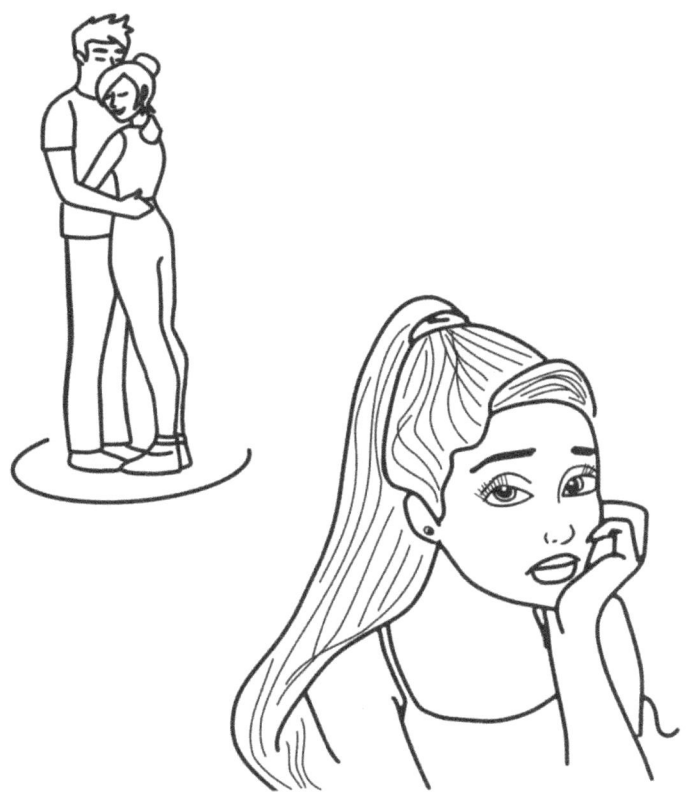

CHAPTER 3

Why don't they choose you?

Not being chosen simply means that you're someone with qualities different from the ones the other person is looking for. Each person chooses the partner or the worker they require, according to their personal or business needs (what they think they need).

I will give you an example related to couples (but it could be applied to any area you choose). The fact that someone doesn't choose you as a partner has nothing to do with you as a person. It has to do with the "need", the other person's taste, what they seek or are familiar with.

Think about the food you like the most, your favorite (the one that makes even you salivate by just thinking about it). Ready? Suppose you thought of a delicious baked pork.

Now I ask you to think about the food that you don't like and that you wouldn't eat at all. Think about it ... Ready? Suppose it's fried fish ... Imagine the best fish, prepared with the best ingredients, by the best chef in the world and served in the best restaurant in your city. They offer you this very fine fried fish or a simple dish of baked pork. Which of the two dishes would you choose? Fried fish or baked pork? Obviously the pork!

If you chose the baked pork, does it mean that the fried fish is "bad?" That it's useless? That it's not worth it? That it's of poor quality? What would the fish say about you choosing the pork?

"Oh, I must be so insignificant, I'm sure I'm worth nothing, that's why they don't choose me". Do you see?

The fact that you've chosen the baked pork has to do with your taste, but nothing to do with the value of the fish itself. Fish may be the best, but it's not what you like. There will be other people who will love the taste of fried fish, and will choose it over any other food. Then, choosing different dishes doesn't have anything to do with the value of each dish. It has to do with everyone's taste or "need".

What are the reasons why they don't choose you?
The fact that they don't choose you has to do with the fact that the person who chooses has "needs" and tastes that are different from you. They are familiar with other types of behavior, of interaction. And they will generally choose what they are familiar with (or the closest to it, whether they like it or not).

Let's imagine that the one who chooses is a woman, whose father is an alcoholic. As much as she hates the behavior of her alcoholic father, she's very likely, among the men who approach her, to end up choosing an alcoholic man.

You may think "But how? Didn't she dislike her dad's alcoholic behavior? It's true, she didn't like it. However, she chooses this behavior because she had to live with her dad all her life. Somehow, she learned to deal with this problem, with this disease. She learned how to handle it. Therefore, even if she doesn't like this situation, she's already familiar with it, and she's very likely to choose a partner who has a drinking problem.

What to do to avoid feeling bad if they don't choose you?
If you have an expectation to be chosen and you aren't, it's natural to feel sad. But it's one thing to feel sad for not having been chosen, and another is to feel that you're worthless because they didn't choose you or because you negatively compare yourself to others. What do I mean by that? I mean, you start thinking "Surely other girls are better than me" or "I'm worth nothing or I'm not enough".

The first thing you have to do is get rid of those negative thoughts. They are just thoughts, not reality. If someone didn't choose you, it's not because you're not good enough, it's because the other person has different "needs" or has a backstory that will lead them to choose people who are more like their father or mother, with behaviors that become more familiar.

Maybe you have a different upbringing or were treated differently. And it's not about you changing to try to please others. The person who loves you will accept you as you are. They will just like you for being original.

Remember, I'm not saying that what he or she is looking for (regarding personal characteristics) is better or worse than what you are or the characteristics you have. I am simply saying that they are different features (not better nor worse, just different).

If I asked you, "Which color is better, red or yellow?" In reality, neither is better nor worse than the other, both are colors. They are simply different.

Some will like red more and others will prefer yellow. It only comes down to taste. Neither one is better than the other.

Once you understand this, you will realize that if someone doesn't *click* with you, it's not because you're not good enough or because you have something bad. It means that your characteristics are different from the characteristics of others this person is familiar with. It has nothing to do with your own worth.

If a particular person doesn't choose you, it doesn't mean that no one is going to choose you. It mean that this person is not the one you would flow with the best. You would flow much better with someone else.

There are many people in the world who could be really compatible and happy with you. As you would be very happy with them too.

So, chin up and allow yourself the opportunity to be pleasantly surprised by life.

Each one will choose according to what they "need" specifically at that moment in their life.

Imagine that someone comes thirsty from the desert". You're the best salty roasted corn, but there is another person who is "contaminated water". Which of the two alternatives do you think the person who comes thirsty from the desert will choose? Obviously the water, without worrying about whether it's contaminated or not. This doesn't mean that this "water" is better than you (the roasted corn). In that moment, the person who comes from the desert needed the water more and that is why he or she chose it.

When you think that you're not good enough for someone,

remember that you're not in competition with anyone. We just all have different qualities. Comparing yourself to others is not a good or accurate strategy.

When you compare yourself to others, you generally do it in a negative way. You see that that the other person is more interesting than you, that they have more beautiful eyes, they are more fun, etc. The truth is that there are always going to be "better and worse" people than you in different areas (qualities, aesthetics, social aspect, etc.). So comparing yourself is not a good idea. You'll waste time and energy.

How to stop feeling something for someone that isn't good for you?

Remember, you deserve the best of the best. If you decide that someone is not good for you, it's because you have realized that there is something (or a lot) in that person that doesn't flow with you, that makes you suffer, that generates pain in you, that takes away more than they give.

Start by loving yourself. By loving yourself you will wish the best for yourself. If you want something that doesn't do you good, think about yourself and try to choose what is best for you.

Suppose you have *diabetes mellitus* and you know that eating sweets could be harmful. You're craving them so you eat some. However, it's not good for you, and you know that you would damage your organs;

So, if you love yourself, even if you really want to eat chocolate, you will avoid it and choose to eat something healthier like vegetables or fruits. That means you choose to eat healthy because you love and take care of yourself. That will give you peace of mind because you'll know that you did something positive for yourself and by yourself. Use this example as an analogy for a romantic or friendship relationship that is not good for you and you decide to end it.

Also, it's not about thinking that you couldn't eat chocolate and keep thinking about the same all day. That can be disturbing. It's about starting to do activities that are really healthy for you and redirecting your mind from the past to the present. Ask yourself, "What else can I do to feel better?" You might think, "I can go to a dance class, for a walk, for a run; I can go for a walk in the park, start painting, start experimenting with clay, I can write a story or I'm going to ride a bike". And you start to do it.

You keep your mind busy with other things. This way, you show yourself that you're important and that if something doesn't suit you, then you leave it and turn around, period. You walk in the opposite direction, encouraged by activities that are fun for you, without looking back. Go ahead and look around you, allow yourself to perceive everything with each of your senses and realize that life or God has other surprises in store for you.

Remember: When one door closes, three doors open. It's about being attentive to those new opportunities that life will bring you. If you don't pay attention, you could walk by and miss the gifts that are meant for you.

In order to receive something new and valuable, you need to leave the old baggage behind. Imagine that someone wants to give you a gold bar, but your hands are busy with "little things" from the past that have no greater value. If you don't let go of those "little things" (resentments, memories that don't help you), you will prevent yourself from hitting the jackpot.

If you let go of everything you carry from the past and keep your heart and mind free, you'll have the opportunity to receive the valuable gifts that life or God wants to give you.

What to do if you have to see someone every day who didn't choose you as a partner?

Each person has the right to choose according to their own needs, requirements or wishes. It doesn't mean they hate you. It's simply that this person cannot offer you what you want.

Suppose the other person is a lemon tree and you're an apple tree. You offer him/her your sweet apples, and you would love for that tree to also offer you sweet apples. However, every time you approach him/her, he/she offers you sour lemons.

You can fertilize the tree, add the best nutrients, take care of it, water it every day. However, despite all your care and everything, it gives you sour lemons again, maybe bigger lemons, but they're acid.

You get upset, you cry and wonder, "Why can't this lemon tree give me sweet apples, like I do?"

What's important here is to realize and accept that they are different. Although both are face to face, in the same garden, no matter what you do, this tree can only give you lemons. It will never give you sweet apples because it's not in its nature.

Once you accept that, you'll stop suffering because the expectation that it could one day give you a sweet apple will disappear. If you're going to stand in front of the lemon tree every day and say: "Why don't you give me apples?" you're wasting your time. You're better off walking through the garden and try to find an apple tree to give you apples.

When you accept that the person you've chosen will not be able to offer you what you want or expect (because it's not in their nature), then you will simply begin to realize the immensity of the garden and you will give yourself the opportunity to continue walking. And perhaps when you stop staring at the lemon tree, you may realize that there are more apple trees to the side or very close to you than you ever imagined (maybe you never saw them). They're waiting for you to discover them and it just depends on you starting to look in another direction. Do you dare to explore?

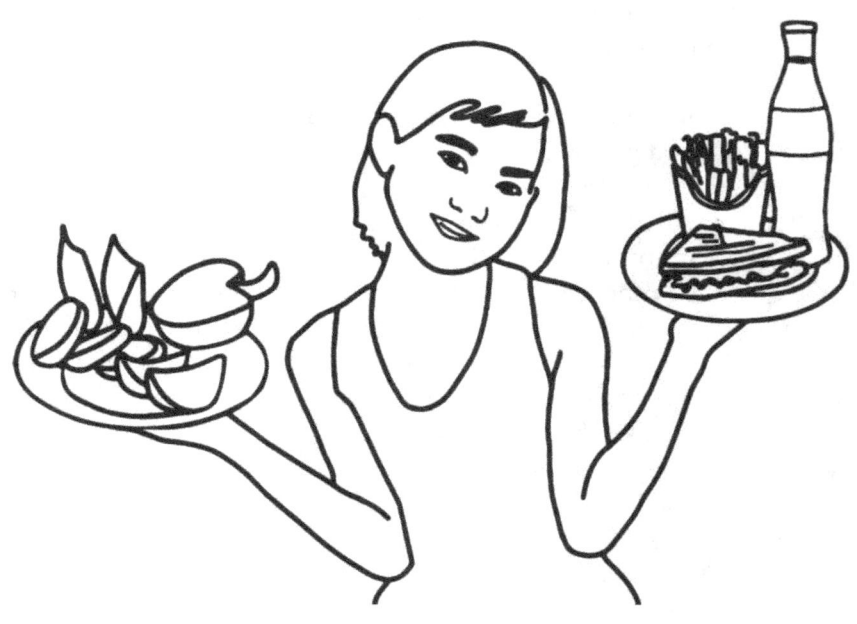

4 You lost your motivation when you lost him/her?

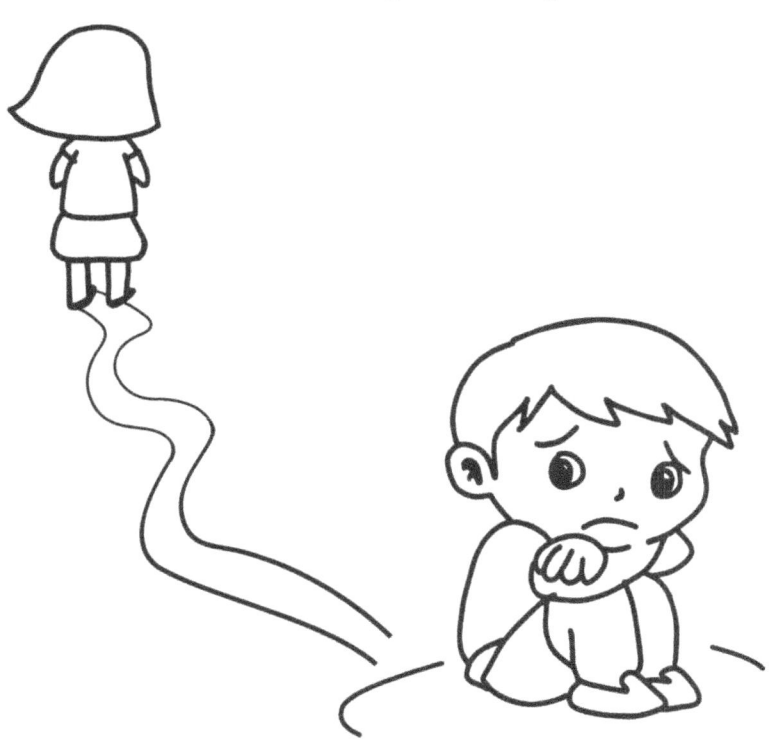

HAVE YOU EVER...?

CHAPTER 4

You lost motivation by losing him/her.

What do you mean by "loss"?

When I speak of "loss", I mean that we no longer have people, situations, or things with us that were meaningful to us. Are they really losses or are they changes?

Thinking of a loss generates pain, sadness, anger, anxiety, frustration. If you can change your outlook and realize that these losses are actually changes that you have to face, the feelings that these changes generate and how you see them could be different.

My father passed away a few years ago. In that moment the pain, the sadness, the wondering why he was gone was inevitable. "Loss" was my first reaction. Sometime later, looking back, I said to myself: "My dad had an illness, he was suffering, but now his spirit has freed himself from the body, from the pain he could have and is at peace", then I thanked God because he was no longer suffering, and that now he enjoys peace. His physical death could be considered as loss or as his birth to a new spiritual life in another dimension. I believe that the spirit remains even after our physical body fades or ceases to exist. I also think that our spirit is energy, and as Lavoisier said: *"Matter is neither created nor destroyed, it only transforms"*.

Therefore, the fact that my daddy was no longer physically among us naturally caused me sadness, nostalgia. But at the same time, I felt comforted and at peace thinking that he had already been born to a new spiritual life, that he now enjoyed the peace of God, without the pain or physical discomfort he endured in life before he passed away.

I remember when my dad came out well after an operation with only a 35% chance of survival, I told him: "Dad, we have to thank God that you're alive!" and he replied: "And even if he was not alive, we must also thank God".

What you call "loss" are actually unexpected changes. They get you out of your comfort zone. A comfort zone is the situation that is familiar to you, that you know, that you've become accustomed to - whether it's pleasant or not - and that you learned to handle in some way.

You call the times you leave your comfort zone "losses" because of that feeling of finding yourself in a different situation, over which you have no control or over which don't know. You find yourself in a different situation and you'll have to learn to adapt. All your adaptation mechanisms will come into play here, in this new situation. So, the so-called "loss" is actually change or not being in your comfort zone.

Why do you lose motivation when you lose someone or something important to you?

First, because something you didn't expect is happening. Let's say you're in shock, you freeze, then you think "This can't be", "Why is this happening to me?" It's difficult to accept that loss, you can feel anger, sadness, anxiety. There can be a whole combination of negative emotions, frustration and all of this, in some way, consumes a lot of your energy.

On the one hand, you miss what's familiar and have a hard time letting go. You don't accept that things have changed, that the person or what you wanted is no longer there. But on the other hand, the healthiest thing is to adapt to this new situation.

When you invest your whole being in someone or something and treat this as something that gives you your own value, when it's gone or when it changes you think that you're worthless, that there is no point in moving on. Any change can generate different emotions, sometimes sadness, sometimes anger, sometimes anguish or anxiety, sometimes a whirlwind of emotions.

The idea is to realize that things have changed, that they are beyond your control, and that it's OK if you cannot control them. You have the necessary resources to go on with your life because it doesn't depend on whether or not a certain person or situation is there, but about what you decide every day and your attitude day by day.

Even when we are all interrelated, each of us has a life of our own. Your reason for life is not someone else's life. Your meaning of life has to do with your dreams, with your expectations, with what you want to contribute to life.

It's normal to miss those who were by your side and have already died. It's important to understand that although they are physically gone, they've simply left their bodies to be born into a spiritual life. And that from this new perspective, in some way, they are with you – they've only been transformed.

Each one has their own story, their own life. Keep building it. Let yourself be positively surprised by life, keep discovering and exploring new moments, the people, the beings that are now with you. We are all travelers in this life. Some have to go before others. As long as we are here, we continue to discover it and forge it. Let's enjoy the moment and the landscapes that we have to share with the other travelers because it's only time we have with them.

It's not about you clinging to someone in particular, it's about sharing intensely with them, the moment you have them close. At the same time, it's important that you learn to keep your hands open and free because the your fellow travelers will get on and off the train unexpectedly.

What to do to regain your motivation and accept the 'loss'?

To accept the loss and regain your motivation, you have to understand that the time of that person, situation or object, ended for you. You have to keep walking (even if you don't have the courage or the strength to do it). Let's go! Get out of bed!

Don't overthink it, just do it! Get up so that you can discover the new things life has for you, and that perhaps will become the best gift you have ever received. Tagore said: "If you cry because the sun has left, the tears will not let you appreciate the beauty of the stars" - and it's so true! Avoid staying stuck in nostalgia, sadness or in the situation of "loss".

It's about accepting that everything has a beginning and an end, and that while you're alive, people, experiences and things close to you will continue to "happen". You just have to watch them to realize that they are there for you! To regain motivation, start doing new things and focus on them.

I'm not telling you to wait until you feel like doing something. Even if you don't feel like it, and it's hard, just start doing it. Even without motivation, when you start to do something, without realizing, you will start to get your motivation back. It's not always from the inside out, sometimes to generate a change or to "re-boost" we start from the outside and it has an impact inside.

A study was carried out where people were hired to work in a company. They were told their shift would be considered completed only if they were very friendly and smiled during the first two hours. So, from 8 to 10 a.m. no matter how they felt they had to smile and be very nice to one another.

All workers were observed to be in good spirits throughout the day. The first two hours were "forced", but the following hours, they naturally felt in a good mood and with a positive attitude. This study showed how change can also happen from the outside in.

The first thing to do to accept **"loss"** is to realize it and accept that whatever you do there is no going back. What's no longer there will never come back.

Imagine you have a glass of milk and it spills into the sink drain. No matter how much you cry, yell and beg, "that" bit of milk will never return to the glass. All that time that you spend yelling and crying over the milk you lost, you could use it in a better way: To accept reality and that you won't be able to change it, to accept that it would be best if you pour yourself another glass of milk. Attention: There is a difference between giving up and accepting a "loss".

Giving up means feeling like a victim in the situation, creating resistance to what happened, immobilizing yourself and "ruminating" on what happened (your thinking remains "hooked" on the situation, going over it time and again). "I already lost Alejandra, I know, but what a shame, why did I lose her? I wish I hadn't. It shouldn't have been like that. I didn't deserve this", and so on. And this way, you keep "ruminating" on what happened.

Accepting has to do with feeling like the protagonist of your life, flowing in the event (that is, not getting stuck in the situation, or keep "ruminating" on it). It means learning from what you've experienced and continuing to walk in a new direction, without extra drama. "I already lost Alejandra. This relationship left me many lessons. Now, I have to keep walking, period".

How to deal with guilt when you lose someone and you didn't go to see them or you think you didn't do enough?

When you do or say something, you do it because at that specific moment you think that it's your best choice in that situation.

Most people don't do or stop doing things with malicious intent. Please stop being unfair to yourself. If in that moment you had foreseen or felt what was going to happen in the future, you probably would've made a different decision. However, with the information you had at that time, in the situation you were going through at that time, you gave an answer or did something according to your possibilities, according to your circumstances or according to the information you had. Nobody stops doing things on purpose to feel guilty afterwards (unless they are a masochist).

What is the difference between guilt and responsibility? Someone is **guilty** when they do things consciously, that is, while they're on their right mind. They do something on purpose (voluntarily and with intent) when they know the consequences of their action.

Someone is **responsible** when they do something without the intent to harm or they're not on their right mind (involuntary and without bad intention), but they harmed someone through their actions.

If you're at next to me when I stretch my arm and I accidentally hit you on the nose, I'm responsible for having hit you, but I'm not guilty. I didn't realize that you were next to me, my hand touched your nose and hit it by accident.

It would be very different than if I was in front of you, I saw you and thought "I want to break your nose" and I hit you hard, with the intention of breaking your nose. There I'd be guilty because I was conscious, on my right mind (without having drunk alcohol for example or without any mental illness) and my intention was really to hit you.

So, when you think that you did not do enough for someone special for you who is no longer by your side, you have to know that you did the best you could at that moment, with the knowledge and understanding that you had in that particular situation - that what you didn't do was not on purpose.

Please understand yourself in that situation. It's not worth it if you keep punishing yourself. You're not a fortune teller, you didn't know what was going to happen. Just know you did the best you could according to your circumstances. After the fact, it's very easy to think "I could've done this", "I could've done that".

If you're totally honest with yourself, you'll realize that the moment you do something, you do it thinking of what is the best thing you can do at that moment.

Most of the time, we act the best way we can, according to our own limitations (not only physical, also personality, health or circumstance factors).

In order to stop feeling guilty about something you did or didn't do, the first thing is to know if you had bad intentions at that moment. Then, when you realize that you didn't act with bad intentions, you'll understand that you're not God or a fortune teller to know what was going to happen, and that at that moment you gave or did the best you could, despite your limitations.

How to handle loneliness?

Loneliness can be lived in peace, joy or pain. You can be surrounded by people and yet feel lonely, or you can be really alone and feel happy and at peace. What does it depend on? On how you feel about yourself, what you're doing and how you value it in that special moment when you're by yourself. It depends on the type of thoughts you may have at that specific moment.

If you feel alone, with or without people around, you're probably having negative thoughts such as "I'm useless", "nobody loves me", "I'm worth nothing", "nobody notices that I'm here", "nobody wants to be with me". Those thoughts are related to negative feelings (sadness, anger, anxiety) and low self-esteem.

You can be alone physically and feel at peace, because you're happy with yourself. You're immersed in your projects, doing activities you like, enjoying the time you have with yourself. You're alone and you enjoy it.

So, being alone is different than feeling lonely.

Feeling lonely is more related to negative thoughts and feelings and low self-esteem. **Being** alone is choosing that time for yourself and keeping busy doing pleasant and fun activities.

How can you overcome an empty heart?

If you feel an emptiness in your heart, it's because you have not yet learned to give yourself affection, love, attention and understanding, but you've probably been looking for it outside: To get it from other people (partner, friends, parents, siblings, etc.).

You can't nurture an empty heart from the outside – it's temporary and you feel good only briefly. Having a full heart has to do with assuming the responsibility and joy of taking care of yourself, of loving yourself, of doing things for you and for yourself because you're important to yourself. It has to do with spending time with yourself to feel better, doing the things that you love. It has to do with congratulating yourself for the positive things you've done. It has to do with being understanding with yourself when you make a mistake, and not with a judgmental attitude that will end up hurting you.

In order to overcome an empty heart, you first need to fill this void with yourself. It means making yourself a priority, taking care of yourself, loving yourself, listening to yourself. With concrete actions, you think about yourself (not only about others, but starting with yourself). In order help other people the best way possible, you first have to be well yourself. And it doesn't mean being selfish.

Some people will wonder if taking care of themselves is selfish or vain. When you spend your time taking care of yourself, you love yourself – it doesn't mean you're vain. Vanity or selfishness would mean that you think only you matter and the rest don't. It would mean getting everything for you and leaving nothing for others.

A full heart means loving, respecting and taking care of yourself first, and then you begin to share the love, peace and knowledge with others around you and that

You're lucky to meet day by day, and with whom you allow yourself to learn, share and teach with simplicity and humility.

How to fill the emotional void?

You fill your emotional void by unconditionally loving and unconditionally accepting yourself, with gratitude for your life, for every apparent quality and shortcoming you may have. Thank God or life for what you are, for what you have or don't have. That speaks of your spiritual growth. It's about filling your life and your heart with love for yourself and with God's love.

From my point of view, spiritual life is very important because whoever has a genuine spiritual life, faces life and its challenges with a more positive and hopeful outlook, with a winning and trusting attitude, despite any difficulty. Because people like that know themselves to be God's children and they know that He is always and will be by their side, that He will never abandon them, that situations that they cannot handle will never touch them and that if they ask for help along the path, the Lord will help them.

I once read a story: A father had asked his seven-year-old son to take some boxes from one place to another. The boy tried with all his might to move the boxes, but he couldn't. He tried and tried, he pushed the boxes but they didn't move half an inch. He insisted with all his might, but nothing worked.

The boy began to feel angry, frustrated, helpless and started crying. He did everything in his power to try to move the boxes and he couldn't do it. Then he approached his father, completely frustrated, crying and said, "Dad, I can't! I can't move the boxes you've asked me to move, just I can't!" The father calmly asked him: "Son, have you done your best to try to move those boxes?" and the son replied: "Yes, I did. I have tried everything!" "Are you sure?" says the father. "Yes, I've tried everything" replied the disappointed child. The father looks at him lovingly, and says: "Son, you haven't tried everything... You haven't asked me to help you move the boxes".

It's important to learn to ask for help, not only from other people, but also from the God you believe in. God respects your freedom so much that he won't intervene in your affairs if you don't ask or don't allow it. And remember that "God is always in your favor, even though it sometimes doesn't seem like it".

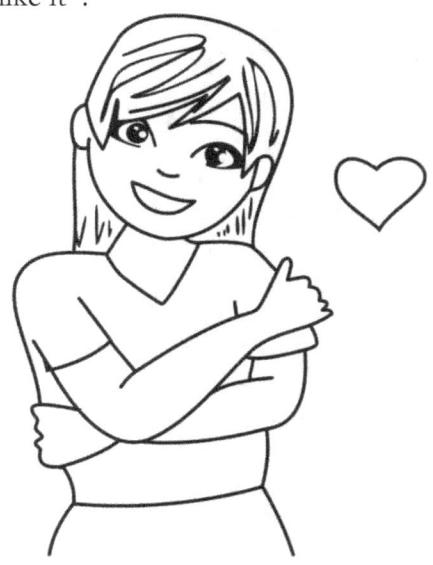

5 How do you free yourself from the past?

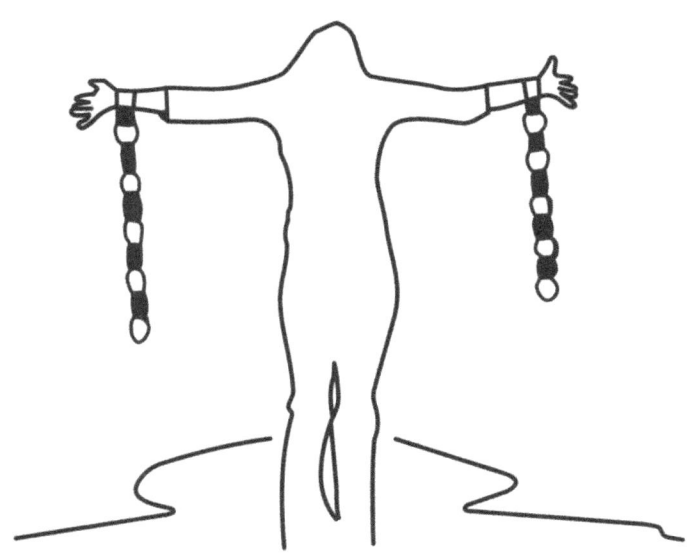

CHAPTER 5
How do you free yourself from the past?

Now we'll talk about how to forget those painful situations that you still keep in your heart. How to let go of past situations that still hurt you.

When we speak of "freeing ourselves", we are implicitly saying that we are stuck or paralyzed by something. When you say, "How do I get rid of the past?" You're saying, "There is something from my past I'm stuck with, something that keeps me paralyzed that I can't get out of my life. It's still there". You still remember it even though it happened in the past.

Specifically, what do you want to free yourself from?

Probably you want to free yourself from those situations that you consider unfair, that caused you pain, anger, concern, feelings of worthlessness, resentment, indignation. Things that you haven't been able to leave behind and continue to carry up to today.

How to free yourself from the past?

Be aware that carrying things from the past into your present will not allow you to move forward. It's as if you were a running motorboat that is tied to the dock. No matter how hard you try to go out to the open sea, if the accelerator is at full throttle, you stay tied to the dock, in the same exact spot.

The pier represents the past and because you're tied there, you don't allow yourself to go to explore the beauties that the open sea has to offer you - all those surprises that you can find, the new places that you can discover if you row ahead on your boat.

In order to free yourself from the past, it's important that you fully live here and now: be fully present today, with all your five senses on.

HAVE YOU EVER...?

The past —with those painful, difficult situations that caused sadness and anger in you— are like unpleasant food that you kept in a suitcase and that you continue to carry until today. If you open that suitcase, a nauseating smell of rotten food that has been stored for weeks, months, years will come out and it will be rotting away everything else you may have in your suitcase, even if they are good things.

Freeing yourself from the past means throwing away all that spoiled food that you keep carrying and getting rid of the suitcase. Why keep holding on to it? Why continue investing energy to keep dragging it if you're not going to use it, if it's not useful or helpful? What for?

And how do you get rid of that suitcase? By experiencing forgiveness. By forgiving yourself, those who hurt you, and the painful situations that you had to experience. In order to free yourself, you need to look at what happened from different angles, from a different perspective, understand the situation from these new points of view, and forgive. Forgiving means letting go. Forgiveness is liberating.

Suppose you prick your finger with a needle and it obviously hurts. Why keep holding the needle in your finger and still feel the pain? You don't need to keep carrying it, you can remove the needle, clean the wound and keep walking. You don't need to keep sticking the needle, let alone leave it stuck there.

When you feel anger, pain or annoyance at being tied to the past and yet you do nothing to free yourself, it's as if you're holding the palm of your hand on a hot iron. Forgiveness means taking your hand off the iron or turning it off so you stop hurting yourself. The act of forgiveness has more to do with you than with the other person. Forgiving and letting go is giving yourself the opportunity to leave pain behind and feel peace again.

Forgiving doesn't mean that you forget what happened. It's not possible because you have a memory and you'll probably remember what happened. However, in order to free yourself from the past it's important that you learn from the painful or difficult situation that you had to endure. Forgiving means saying to yourself: "This happened to me that I didn't like.

What do I learn from this situation and what will I do differently next time?" Once you learn and are clear about what you'll do differently, the next time something similar happens to you, you can let go of the past and stop thinking about it. You just keep the lesson, what you learned and what you're going to do differently next time. You let go of the rest, you let it go out of your life and of your memory.

Alexia is a dermatologist. During the COVID pandemic, she worked remotely and gave appointments to each one of her patients at a specific time. One of per patients, Janet, usually showed up on time for her appointments. One day they met at 4:00 p.m., but it was 4:15 p.m. and Janet hadn't logged on. Alexia got worried because Janet was usually on time.

She called her and when Janet answered, she reacted aggressively towards Alexia, and told her: "Why are you calling me, if we already agreed I was going to connect at four?" And she kept talking to her in a very agitated and annoyed way. Alexia didn't understand Janet's reaction.

She had only called her because she was worried about her, because her being late was unusual. Janet told her: "I'll be online for my appointment in a bit, so don't call me again". That situation was uncomfortable for Alexia. She felt hurt because she had been worried about her patient and that is why she called her. However, apparently her patient, Janet, felt it as if Alexia was trying to control her.

I asked Alexia" "What did you learn from this situation with your patient Janet? She said: "I learned that next time, if this patient (Janet) specifically takes a long time logging on for her appointment, I won't call her, not because I'm angry about her reaction with me but because I understood that her way of handling things is different from mine. And that even when I act in good faith, I could be misunderstood.

So to avoid misinterpretations, I prefer simply not to call her, even when she is late for her appointment. And so, Alexia forgot about this matter in her mind and in her heart. Another important thing to free yourself from the past is that you can say exactly what bothered you.

Learn to have "closure": To not be left with something pending to say to a person. Tell them what bothers you, express it right then and in an appropriate way or whenever you are able to. Discuss it directly with the person you had the problem with.

If for some reason you couldn't or didn't have the opportunity to discuss it with the person involved, you can do what I call "closure from the couch". What does it mean? It means you can visualize, in a relaxed state, a guided conversation with this person and you can close the chapter through this method, drop it and let it go of your life.

As you can see, "closure" doesn't necessarily have to happen in the presence of the person you had the conflict with. There are different ways to "close" painful situations and let them go, but to stay at peace the essential thing is to learn the lesson. Say: What will I do differently next time I'm in this kind of situation? It is important that you remember what you have learned, because if you don't, you'll learn the hard way by repeating the pattern.

You start to feel pain when you're under pressure. When you feel that your most sensitive side is exposed. No matter how light someone touches your wound, it will hurt you because it has pus inside, right?

The first thing you have to do is locate in what situation, in what time, with whom those negative things happened to you or that hurt you and that you simply kept in and didn't want to know about or remember. Once you locate the emotional wounds, you begin to clean them, to understand what happened, gently, until you puncture them. What does it mean?

To locate what exactly hurt you so much. Then you start working on the ideas that come to mind, the beliefs you have, then you replace them with more positive ones or to learn the lesson from what you've experienced. What does that mean? Be aware of what you've taken away from that painful situation.

For example, "Okay, this happened to me, so what lesson has this difficult situation taught me? What did I learn?" and you immediately ask yourself: "What will I do differently next time I'm in a similar situation?" Then you say: "What I'll do differently is…", "Before I reacted like this, but the next time it happens to me, I'll respond this way".

Once you draw the conclusion (what you'll do differently next time thanks to the lesson you learned), you can let the situation that hurt you out of your life. You let it go and forget about it for good because you've learned your lesson.

If you do the process right, it will stop hurting (remember, it's not overnight but it works).

If you don't learn the lesson, the "torture" will continue, as if to say, "I'll stay here until you learn what I came to teach you". When you say: "I learned this and next time I'll do this differently", then you will have removed all the accumulated pus and the wound will heal.

If you don't locate the things that you still have accumulated, you could end up like those people who have emotional pain and unconsciously look for very sad novels or movies, to give themselves permission to cry for the situation that really hurts them. Those movies are just an excuse to cry.

Technique to free yourself from recurring thoughts.
This is a technique that will help you free yourself from those thoughts that come and go, those thoughts that every time you start to do something, boom! They pop up! And you can't stop thinking about them. It's a very effective and simple technique, I invite you to try it.

When you can't stop thinking about something or if intrusive thoughts pop up while you're doing your activities, and you feel "invaded" by them, it's important that you fix a certain time during the day (for example, ten minutes) to think about that topic or person that comes to your mind throughout the day.

Let's say you decide: "I'm going to think about this situation at 8:00 p.m. for ten minutes". So, if during the day, a thought referring to that situation that bothers you pops up, as soon as it appears, you immediately tell yourself: "I'm going to think about this at 8:00 p.m." and you go about your day.

Apply this technique throughout the day. Whenever an intrusive thought pops up about what's bothering you, tell yourself: "I'm going to think this at 8:00 p.m." and you "postpone" it for that hour. The thought will remain "calm".

It won't insist because it knows that you're going to give it attention at a certain time. And when the time comes, you'll really dedicate those ten minutes to think about it. What you didn't think of at that time or you forgot and then you remember, will be thought about at your scheduled time the next day. That way, you'll free your whole day of those thoughts that didn't leave you alone or tortured you.

The thought stops "insisting" when it knows that you are going to give it a time slot. It is like a child who insists you give him chocolate cake. If you say: "Look, I'm going to give you the chocolate cake, at certain time, after dinner". It is very likely that the child will stop insisting, because he already knows what time you will give it to him. But if you don't say anything or if you simply say "don't bother me", the child will come back and insist until you pay attention to him. However, when you set a specific time, and you assure the child that you will give him the chocolate at that time, he will remain calm.

Thoughts work the same way. If you give it a specific time each time it "bothers" you, you simply remind it, "I will think about that issue at certain time". That way, the thought will stop bothering you throughout the day. Doing that won't take more than a few seconds.

How to overcome negative experiences?

It depends on how and what you're feeding your thoughts with. If you want to forget those negative experiences, one of the main steps is to forgive, whether you have to forgive yourself or others. It's about letting go of the situation. It's about knowing that all of us, as human beings, can get it right or make mistakes that the reaction you have is up to you. And how the other person reacts, that depends and speaks of them. Remember that each one gives according to who they are or what they have.

If that person is a source of contaminated water, they will offer you just that: contaminated water. If you're someone who offers flowers, then the perfume will remain in your hands, and in the hands of those who receive that perfume. Each one gives based on what they are, based on what they have or what they do. What the other person does speaks of them, what you do speaks of you.

Anyone can make a mistake, and doesn't deserve to be judged for that. It's not about judging others because we can all make mistakes. As Jesus said: "He that is without sin, let him cast the first stone". It's all about understanding, not about judging.

Another way to overcome negative experiences is to reflect, to do something positive to compensate for the negative that you could have done. If someone did something negative against you, you have to put yourself in a position to forgive because that person probably has a lot of pain in their life (or probably may have a disease you do not know of) and expresses it through their actions.

Remember that everyone will give according to who they are. What will a floral perfume give? Floral perfume, obviously. Now imagine a pile of garbage, what will emanate? The smell of garbage, and not only for you, but for each person who deals with it.

What to do so that the memory of hurtful words stops hurting?

Sometimes there are hurtful words that are really hard to forget. A technique that can help neutralize the negative impact that those words left on you is to imagine that they are pronounced with a tone of voice that is funny to you or that makes you laugh. For example, the technique has worked very well for me using the voice of Donald Duck or Porky Pig. Then you imagine that those hurtful words are said with that same funny voice, coming from your foot, and after listening to them, you kick them out of your life.

How to heal emotional wounds?

Stop remembering those things that hurt you. Drop that bag of knives you keep carrying and that keeps hurting you. Forgive those painful situations, forgive yourself for what you're punishing yourself for even now. Forgive other people's reactions, words, actions, or omissions. Stop idealizing people or situations and see them as they really are.

Accept reality, understand that things are the way they are, not how you want them to be. In other words, learn to handle the disappointment or frustration that you bring on yourself when things don't go the way you want or when you want.

Healing emotional wounds has a lot to do with forgiveness, with the realization that each one gives based on what they are and on what they can give, from their life experiences, from the teachings or how they were treated, from the situations they were going through at a certain time.

Have you ever judged others just based on the little bit you know about a situation? Have you ever judged even when you don't have the full picture, but you still judge, make mistakes and save the situation that hurt you without asking, with all the assumptions you made at that specific moment?

When you make an assumption, the first five will be a negative one out of ten assumptions. Many times you feel hurt due to things that were not really happening, but you assumed they were. Another important way to heal emotional wounds is by clarifying the situation. What does it mean to clarify? It means to get information, to ask to and find out. Go ask the source directly, if possible, in order to understand why things happened in a certain way. Don't assume or believe that you already know the answer, but go as the source up front.

And if you no longer have the opportunity to talk with the source, then understand that there are certain reasons for people to react in one way or another, not necessarily with the goal to harm you. It can also be due to the person's ignorance or their lack of knowledge regarding values. It's important to understand that others are not your clones, that they won't act as you would, that they won't think as you would, that they won't have the gestures that you would have, that they may not have your intelligence. Therefore, their reactions are going to be diametrically opposite to the way you would go about things.

You're likely wondering how is it possible that this person treats me this way, if I was only positive towards that person? Well, everyone gives what they have. You can suddenly be a loving, affectionate cat and perhaps the other person is a hedgehog.

Probably you approach them with the greatest affection to hug them, and the only thing that person will do is prick you with their quills, not because they're bad, but because it's their nature: their body is covered with quills. They didn't pinch you to intentionally hurt you. You approached them, and pricked yourself with something that was natural to it.

The intention in every action is essential to understand what happens to you. If your emotional wounds were caused by someone who did something to you "with malicious intent", first think about whether or not it's your assumption. If this person acted with bad intentions towards you, please be compassionate, think how great their pain must be that all they do is try to hurt others.

A person who feels too hurt is probably going to be hurtful. Someone whose self-esteem is on the ground is probably going to be the one who reacts aggressively, because that's the only way they feel superior to you.

Emotional wounds are also caused by those situations that didn't meet your expectations. Deep down, could it be that your ego got hurt? And if so, is it worth it to keep your ego suffering?

You will heal your emotional wounds by forgiving and understanding that nobody is perfect, that we can all make mistakes, that each one gives according to what they have and who they are, based on their life experiences. You need to understand that by bringing painful things from your past to the present, all you do is continue on the trail of sorrow in your present. You must understand that you're wasting time and energy investing in things from the past that are no longer here, but that you're "bringing them back to life" in the present.

Emotional wounds occur because things had a negative outcome, which you didn't expect. Now in the present, you can build a new life, you can redirect your energy and channel it towards those situations that will add to your life and will be more positive for you.

Instead of wasting your time and energy thinking about negative things, invest it in building and doing things that you enjoy, learn new things, explore new activities – explore life!

Four steps to free yourself from the past:
1. - Place yourself 100% in the present, with all your senses.
2. - Forgive.
3. - Take the lesson out of that situation and let it go.

Letting go of the situation means not returning to it to think or talk about it. Get it out of your mind and your words. In other words, stop repeating it in your mind and stop telling others. Just leave it where it's at, where it happened: in the past. What do you keep? With the present and with the lesson you learned from that situation, focus your attention on your present activity and your day to day.

4. - Start new activities that require all your focus because if you already know them, you'll do them mechanically. And the true goal of all this is to reorient your thinking and your focus on new opportunities and interests to keep your mind busy with your full attention.

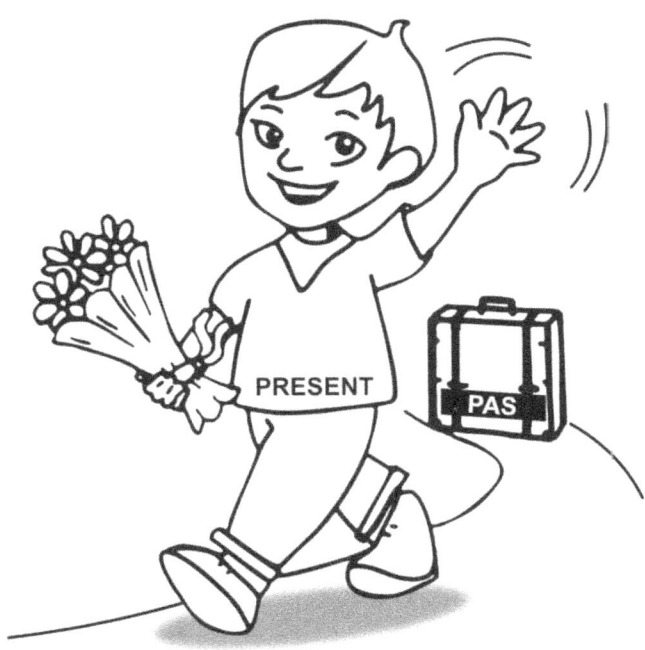

HAVE YOU EVER...?

6 IT'S HARD FOR YOU TO TAKE ACTION

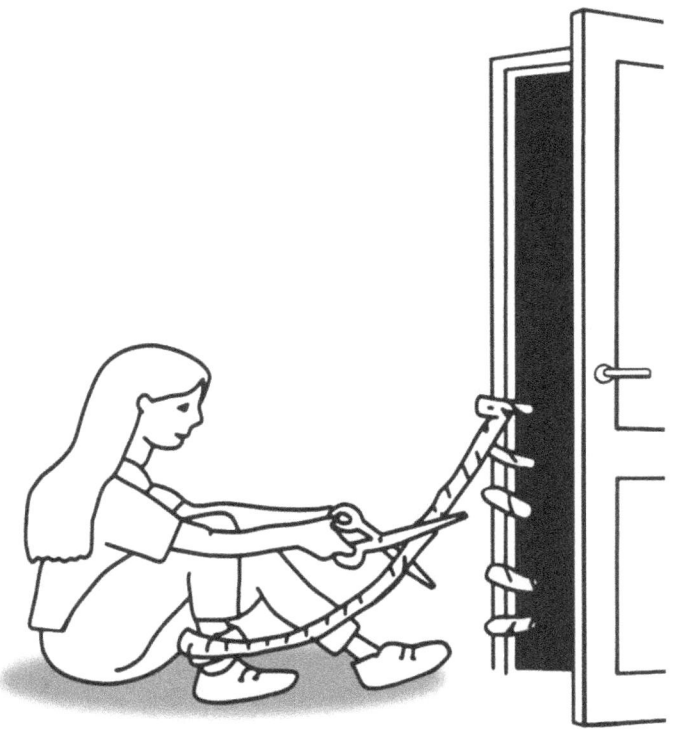

HAVE YOU EVER…?

CHAPTER 6
It's hard for you to take action.

What does "taking action" mean?

It means starting to turn ideas or pending issues into concrete actions. It's making what you think, what you imagine, what you want come true. It may not happen quickly, but it's possible and easier than you imagine.

Why is it difficult for you to take action?

It could be for different reasons. First, because you don't feel capable (due to lack of skills or knowledge). Second, for fear that if you fail, others will make fun of you (or that you'll "disappoint" yourself), for fear that a good outcome would bring you greater responsibilities. Maybe if you do it right, next time it would have to be the same or better. Laziness is also an obstacle because you see that it's something too ambitious or big and you think that you won't be able to finish it.

How to start taking action?

Once you have an idea of what you want to do, you just have to do it, without overthinking – just do it. Years ago, I worked at a hospital. My house was about twenty minutes away and I had a friend who lived about an hour away. We had to start 8:00 a.m. and usually I would arrive at 7:55 a.m. or 8:00 o'clock at the latest. But my friend who lived an hour away would always arrive half an hour earlier.

I knew that because during my night shifts, I would see her arrive at around 7:20 a.m. or 7:30 a.m. at the latest.

One day I told her: "You live one hour from the hospital and you always arrive at 7:15 or 7:30 a.m. I live twenty minutes away and I usually arrive just on time. Don't you feel lazy getting up so early so you can get to the hospital half an hour earlier?" She told me: "Of course I do". So, I said: "How do you get up and come so early?"

And my friend shared her secret with me: "Look, I set my alarm clock at 5:30 a.m. and when it rings, I don't even think about it, I jump out of bed and go shower, because if I keep thinking I won't get up". So I realized that the secret was simply doing it. I wanted to try it, the next day I set my alarm at 6:30 a.m. and as soon as the alarm went off, I didn't even think about it, I jumped out of bed, went to shower and, indeed, I arrived at work early! I have applied this same technique to other situations and it works with unquestionable success. If, for example, I want to clean and tidy up my desk, instead of thinking, "I'm going to tidy up my desk, first I'll remove everything, then I'll start cleaning each part of the desk. Then, I'll do this and that", I simply take action, I start tidying up (without thinking). That way I have good results, I move much faster than I can imagine and I finish things sooner than planned. If I had thought about every step I was going to take, I would have gotten tired even before I started doing something and I wouldn't have done it.

You want to start something and you don't.

You have the desire to do something and you probably don't do it because it seems complicated or you think you'll have to make a big effort to achieve it, then unconsciously you avoid it and start doing other "important" things because maybe they seem easier or shorter to complete.

Other times, you feel that you lack information or knowledge to do something. When you have those doubts and you don't feel capable, you unconsciously start to sabotage yourself and prioritize other types of activities, while you're ignoring what you really wanted to do.

How to specify what you would like to do?

The first thing is that you're clear about what you want to do in a general and specific way. You need to know where you want to go, what is your destination and what you want to achieve. Just keep in mind that to achieve what you want, you don't need to have an exact path to reach that destination. You don't need to know every step you're going to take to achieve your specific goal.

Second, instead of stalling in all the planning, when you already know where you want to go, simply start walking and as you go you see what you need to do and you keep going forward. You go forward and you do. You do and you go forward, without stopping too much to think. All you have to do to take action is to start doing it.

I'm not saying you have to wait for the moment when you feel ready to start, because the reality is you're never going to feel ready. So, as soon as you've thought about what you want to do, just simply start doing it, take action, stop waiting for "the perfect moment" because it doesn't exist. You're going to create the right moment with your small daily actions and those little steps will be the ones that will bring you closer to what you want.

If you set yourself a goal that seems "too big", that very idea can scare you and paralyze you in such a way that you don't even try to take the first steps. What's the solution? When the goal is "too big" (real or apparently), you just need to divide it into smaller goals and in turn, divide these smaller goals into even smaller ones.

If, for example, someone told you "You have to eat this cow", you'll most likely think: "I won't be able to" and you wouldn't even try. But if you cut this cow into pieces and each piece was divided into smaller ones, you'll likely start eating those small pieces. Then, without realizing it, little by little you'll end up eating the whole cow.

As you can see, it's about taking small steps towards your goal. Divide the big goal into smaller goals and if those goals still seem big to you, shrink them a little more, until they are achievable for you. And so, step by step, go forward until you reach the goal you set for yourself. I remember I had a 72-year-old patient, Juanita, whose cardiologist had told her to walk one hour a day. Her husband, Raúl, who was with her that day during our appointment, told me that Juanita didn't want to walk. She said: "Doctor, I won't be able to".

This was a sedentary woman who didn't do much physical activity. Imagine what it meant for someone like that to have to walk an hour a day. It was "too big" of a goal for her.

So, I asked Juanita, "Do you think you can walk inside your apartment for a minute, every day, with a watch?" and she said,

"Ahhh... one minute every day, yes, that I can do. One minute a day!? Sure!" And so she began to walk one minute a day for a week. At the next appointment, a week later, I suggested walking three minutes a day and she did. The following week, it was five minutes a day. And so, Juanita started the habit of walking daily. Finally, by her own decision, she began to walk for fifteen minutes, then thirty until she started walking an hour daily, next to her husband and in the park in front of her house.

Let me tell you, something similar happened to me. I wanted to walk on the treadmill I have on the third floor at home, but I honestly felt lazy. Then, I thought: "I'll do it like Juanita, who walked a minute a day at the beginning", but to tell you the truth, I procrastinated. So I said to myself: "Suddenly walking for a minute is still too big a goal for me, so I'm going to narrow the goal and start by going up to the third floor of my house and looking at the treadmill", and I did so for a week. The following week, I said, "very well, now I'm going to the treadmill and will stay on it for a few seconds". And that's how it was.

I went up to the third floor, I stood on the machine, without turning it on, and I stayed there for about 30 seconds. The following week, I said to myself "Well, it's time to turn on the machine and start walking, even for a minute", and I turned on the treadmill, I started walking and it was not one minute but fifteen. So I increased the time until I could walk one hour every day. Very good, Susy! Mission accomplished!

You worry about what may happen.

"Pre-occupying" doesn't help you to take action. You anticipate the future by giving it a negative or catastrophic look, you assume what will happen, and you consider it a certainty (as if that were really the only possible reality and that it will definitely happen). Has it ever happened to you? Does it sound familiar to you?

35 years ago, people communicated through hand-written letters. Cell phones didn't exist, nor the internet. So, when a person was going to work in another country, let's say someone from Peru was going to work in Japan, people would say: "Oh, what a shame!" Because a letter would take a month to get from Peru to Japan, and we had to wait another month to receive a reply (if they answered immediately). Parents who thought about their children who

travelled to Japan to work felt very sad because they thought that they wouldn't be able to communicate with them often because international phone calls were too expensive at that time.

If 35 years ago, a mother gave birth to a child and thought "when my son grows up, if he goes to Japan to work when he is 18 years old, I'll suffer a lot because I'll hardly be able to communicate with him", that mother would have been suffering in vain and in advance because cell phones and the internet came along in the following years. And if that son was eighteen years old at this time and travelled to Japan to work, he could certainly communicate in real time and see his mother or anyone on the screen, anywhere in the world.

Thirty years ago, that technological evolution was only a dream, now it's a reality. Then, that mother who thought, "If my son goes to work in Japan, I'll suffer a lot because I'll have to wait too long to communicate with him", would have suffered in vain due to an assumption because many things have changed since then.

It's like being in the middle of summer and you meet a friend who is dressed in a long-sleeved sweatshirt, jacket, coat, gloves, woollen socks and hat. You ask him "What are you doing dressed like this in the middle of summer?" "Aren't you hot?" And he tells you: "Of course I'm hot! But what if winter comes? I'd rather be prepared..." What would you make of this situation?

You have to live each thing at its own time, neither before nor after, at the exact moment when you have to experience it.

How do you face the fear of what could happen, but hasn't happened yet?

Thoughts are just that: thoughts, assumptions. They're not evidence or reality, at least until they're proven with concrete facts. The fact that you think that something can happen doesn't mean that it will definitely happen, it's only a possibility in a million possibilities.

Whenever you think negatively, open the range of possibilities to more positive ones. Just as it's possible for things to happen in a negative way, it's also possible for things to happen in a positive or similar way. It's not just black or white, there are a thousand possible shades.

For example, if you say "If I go to the store, most likely won't find these candies I'm looking for", it's true, it could happen. What other possibilities are there? You will likely find these candies at the store.

Maybe on the way, you'll find another store, where you can find the candies you're looking for. "It's possible that someone will come to my house and bring you the candy you want as a gift". You have to open up to the range of possibilities.

Another example: You and a friend agree to meet at 4:00 p.m. but its 5:00 and she hasn't arrived or called.

Your first thought could be: "She must've forgotten we were meeting today" or "She wasn't interested in meeting me". They are negative thoughts or assumptions, but they're not necessarily true. What other possibilities are there?

Maybe she lost her wallet and didn't have money to move on her to get to where you were. Another possibility is that she lost her cell phone or an emergency arose and she couldn't let you know you, etc.

What do you do with all these assumptions? Go to the source and ask your friend, "Hey, we had a meeting at 4:00, I've been waiting for you an hour ago, what happened?" She will give you a concrete answer. By asking her directly, you can stop doubting and guessing.

The assumptions also prevent you from taking action because the famous "What if...?" comes to mind. (What if I do not succeed? What if things are not as I think? What if my calculations are wrong? ...). Remember that the "What if ...?" is also an assumption, it doesn't exist, you can delete it or remove it from your vocabulary.

How to stop assuming?

Start by asking, by looking at the evidence. When you assume, you're interpreting things according to your point of view. Just because it's on your mind, it means that it's the truth.

A man was driving on the road, he hits a curve and sees a woman driving in the opposite direction. .Then the man rolls down the window and yells, "Cow!" and the lady responds, "idiot!" and when she turns the curve, she bumps into a cow.

What happened? The lady thought the man was insulting her and that is why she replied with another insult. However, when the man yelled "cow" at her, he only wanted to warn her that there was a cow crossing up ahead. He wanted to warn her. She had assumed that the man was insulting her. See how an assumption can show you a totally different picture than it really is. And that assumed scenario can lead you to have an inappropriate or even dangerous reaction (like what happened with the cow).

How to overcome negative emotions to go after what you want?

To avoid negative emotions (distrust, insecurity, fear, etc.), you can start by trusting that you're going to do things in the best possible way for yourself. What you'll do doesn't have to be perfect, just relax and enjoy what you're doing. Just be ready and do it with the best intention.

Let go and flow (without pressure, without judgment). When you do things this way, the results are usually positive because you're doing it truly from your heart.

It's normal to feel fear when you want to do something new. But remember that fears are thoughts too and you can get rid of them. How? Just by looking at the situation from another angle, seeing the positive side of things. Knowing that nobody is asking you for perfect results, but for you to do things in the best possible way, calm, relaxed, and enjoying what you do.

Believe in yourself, that you're capable of getting positive results (it doesn't matter if you failed a little or a lot before). Give yourself the opportunity to have more confidence in yourself. Remember, there is no one right way to do things. We can have positive results doing things one way or another. There is no single way to obtain the desired or expected results.

You don't need to be an expert to do something. We are all learning along the way, we're not born knowing. Life is a constant learning process. I like to say that we are "learners in progress" every one of us. Doing something is simply taking a step, leaving the place where you're parked in order to move forward. It doesn't matter that you move half an inch, what matters is that you're leaving that spot you were parked at (like Juanita, who started walking for a minute a day).

You're moving forward! Nobody is asking you to do it at lightning speed. Just take the step (even if it's a baby step). The important thing is to keep moving forward with a positive attitude, without judging yourself, without criticizing yourself - rather understanding and supporting yourself.

Your brain knows it, but you do the opposite... Why?

When you rationally know that something is positive, but do the opposite, you're most likely sabotaging yourself. You consciously want to achieve something, but inside (on an emotional and/or subconscious level) there is some fear or a greater need that you're not seeing, and that is distracting you from your rational goal.

You have to discover that "not doing" what you apparently want to do. What is it saving you from? What is it protecting you from?

Ricardo had made great efforts to come to Lima from Arequipa, to be hired by a prestigious company. He obtained the position as a commercial manager. During the first year, he showed exceptional performance: he was punctual, he adequately solved any challenge, and he was leading the company's growth in a very positive way. But during his second year, this young manager started to arrive late, he didn't fulfill his assigned tasks and the company's owner, realizing his drastic change, sent him to therapy.

Ricardo's girlfriend, Leslie, in Arequipa. He missed her, he wanted to go back and be with her. He wasn't "aware" that this was the real reason why his job performance had plummeted. We discovered it over a few sessions.

You might think, why didn't he just ask permission or quit and go to Arequipa? Ricardo had come to Lima with her mother, they came from a lower-middle class family, and he was afraid of disappointing his mom by saying: "I want to go to Arequipa because I miss my girlfriend a lot and I want to spend more time with her".

How would his mother have reacted if he had told her, "Mom, I have resigned from this great position of commercial manager in Lima, because I miss Leslie who is in Arequipa?"

His mom would have been up in arms (she would have probably been mad at him). But if they had fired him, it would have been easier for him to say: "Mom, they fired me. It's better if we return to Arequipa, I'll look for another job there". His mom would have said, "Yes, honey, let's go back home. There, we'll see find opportunities". Ricardo's greatest need was to go back to Arequipa because he missed his girlfriend. He liked his job, but his greater need made him sabotage his job. And you, have you ever wanted to do something and did exactly the opposite?

When one part of you says "I should do this" and the other part says, "But I want to do something else", the decision you finally make, to do or not to do, is related to your greatest need, i.e., to what that is most valuable or important to you. If you look back, you realize that you took certain steps because they gave you that thing that was valuable or important to you.

What is self-sabotage? It is you planning to do something and you end up doing the opposite or different from what you supposedly want or what would lead you to fulfill your apparent goal because deep down there is something else more important or valuable for you. For example, I want to read this book, but I have to clean the kitchen, I have to sort my things, I have a thousand "important" and justifiable things to do.

It also usually happens when you want to do something or make progress in a project and remember other important things that you have to do, you prioritize the latter because it's easier to say, "I'm not making progress with my project because I have to do this important thing". Somehow, you look good or better with yourself, than saying, "I'm not doing my project because I'm lazy or I don't feel like doing it".

Let's say you have a business meeting at the office at 5:00 p.m. and suddenly, half an hour before, you start having a terrible headache. What happened here? It's much easier to say: "I'm not going to my work meeting because I have a terrible headache" than to say to yourself, "I'm not going to work meeting because I don't feel like it or because I'm bored or I just don't want to go".

Then unconsciously, more often than not your body can generate physical discomforts – that you actually feel – even if your body feels well. It's a way to "self-justify" and to look good with yourself, not just with others. This way, it's easier not to accept having done the activity you had planned (and I'm not saying that "all" headaches are due to this).

You doubt yourself a lot… Will you be able to do this?

I think that nobody feels completely prepared to do something. Every now and then that fear creeps in, the question of whether we'll be able to do something the way we want to. What we have to learn is to give the best of ourselves, regardless of the final outcome.

It's about knowing that when doing something, you gave the best of yourself. Understanding the circumstances in which you found yourself and the context where the situation occurred. Whether something happens or not, in one way or another, not only depends on you but on many circumstances and situations. So this is simply about putting your best foot forward with the best attitude, regardless of the end result.

Keep on your mind that that you gave your best, and enjoyed what you did. It's not about perfect results. Maybe they aren't and that's OK because perfect is the enemy of good. When you have a perfectionist attitude, you miss out on the small beautiful details. Perfectionism even takes away spontaneity in certain activities.

The important thing is that you give the best in what you do and leave the final outcome in Life's hands. Remember that the final results won't speak of your ability in itself, but of how all the circumstances came together and your effort to do what you wanted to do.

If you don't do it, someone else will ... Right?

It's true. If you don't do certain thing, someone else can do it, but they won't do it as you would, with the experience that you have. Suppose you're asked to make a free painting on a wall that will decorate a street in your neighborhood.

Suddenly, you think, "I'm not that good, someone else should do it". And that's fine, maybe someone else will do the drawing, but the image I put on that wall won't have the same characteristics of the image you would have created. It just won't be as you would've done it. It probably won't use the same colors that you would have used. So, yes, something can be done, but it won't ever be the way you would've done it – You are unique.

When something is asked of you, or when life gives you the opportunity to do something, it's because nobody like you will do it the way you would and perhaps it is your way of doing things that is required. To generate a certain impact or have a certain outcome that someone else won't have, even if they do a job similar to yours. Remember, you are unique.

How do you motivate yourself to get up even though you physically don't want to?

Don't think about it, just do it. This is not about whether or not you feel like getting up or doing things. It's about you starting to do it, without overthinking.

How do I get up when I don't want to? Just stop thinking so much and act. Just by doing, you will motivate yourself to continue moving forward. If you stay lying in bed, you'll tend to continue like this. If you think about it too much, you won't get up. The only way to get up is to just get up and do it, without overthinking.

Usually what stops you is the ideas, not the reality. You have the belief that you're not going to like something, without having tried it, and you say that you don't like it.

Camila used to say, "What am I going to cook? I'm not good at cooking". However, the truth is that she had never tried. With the unfortunate COVID-19 pandemic, Camila remained in quarantine at home, and the lady who helped her had to stop working.

Since Camila didn't cook and had to eat, she started looking for recipes, she started doing trial and error and I remember her telling me that one day, she wanted to make an omelette.

She needs to separate the yolk from the egg white, and to achieve an "acceptable" result (without the yolk breaking), she ended up breaking eight eggs.

Many will say: "She had to break eight eggs to separate a yolk from a white without damaging the yolk?" Yes, and the moment she did it, she literally jumped of joy and congratulated herself for having achieved it. The second time she did it, she no longer had to break eight eggs. She only broke three eggs and she was happy because she broke her own record.

Anyone would say "what a shame". But actually Camila felt happy because she made progress in what was difficult for her. It was something that she hadn't done before, and yet, thanks to her perseverance, she was able to achieve it. She also found cooking relaxing and fun.

"I'm not necessarily saying that my dishes are perfect or delicious, just that cooking relaxes me and that the meals I make taste delicious", she told me. So those ideas of "I'm not good at cooking" or "I don't like cooking" vanished the moment Camila started cooking.

One day a very dear friend, Gaby, called me to go to a bonsai class. To tell you the truth, I'm not really a plant lover and I've never really worked on the garden. I agreed to go along with her not only because I enjoy her company, but also because she wanted to experiment, explore something new (I had never made bonsai). And much to my surprise, I really enjoyed that class and had a great time.

The idea of attending a bonsai class didn't bring me the greatest joy (to be totally honest). However, once I started the class, I felt really happy and I discovered that it was a pleasant activity that connected me with life, from another angle.

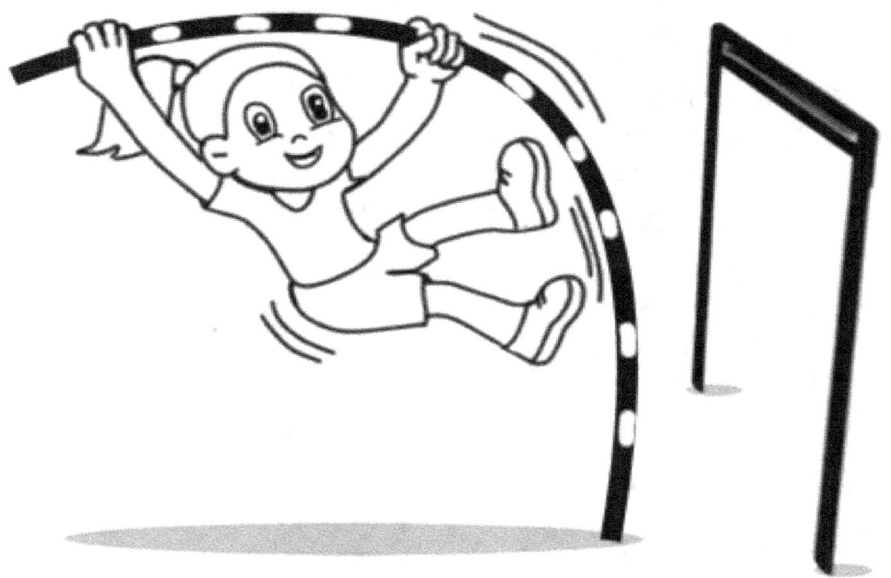

7 How to keep a positive attitude in difcult situations?

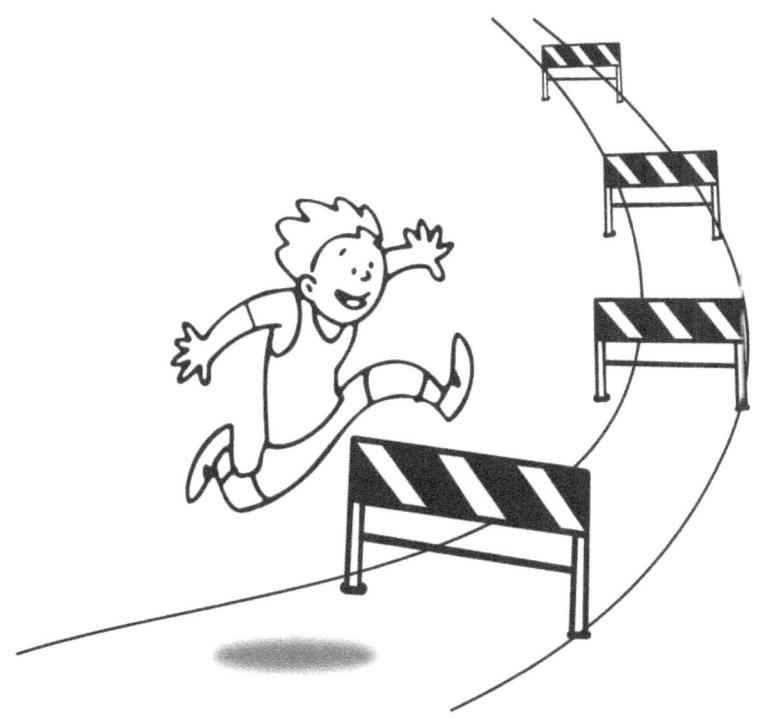

HAVE YOU EVER…?

CHAPTER 7
How to keep a positive attitude in difficult situations?

What is a positive attitude?

It means looking at the situation objectively, focusing on its favorable side; looking at what adds up, what you can learn, what the situation teaches you, expecting the best of it and maintaining your best attitude to face it. That's what it is to have a positive attitude.

How can you stay positive when your world is "falling apart"?

It has to do with knowing that everything that happens to you is for something positive in your life, and that what happens to you is nothing more than what you're capable of coping with.

God or life will never put you in situations you can't face, but if you have had to live a certain situation it's because you're able to face it positively. Everything could crumble down, but as long as you're alive, you'll be able to get ahead. Look, for you to be conceived, an egg and a sperm had to come together.

But before fertilization occurred, the ovum was surrounded by millions of spermatozoa and only the most capable one, the most skilled, was the one that managed to penetrate the ovum and fertilize it. And that's where you come from – that skillful sperm. You're the best of nature, in that time and place.

You come from the most skilled, the most capable and intelligent sperm, the one that reached the goal first. So, from your origins, you're a champion, you're a fighter, someone capable of getting to the finish line successfully.

HAVE YOU EVER...?

Remember this to keep a positive attitude, from the time of your conception you're the best of the best. You're a human being with qualities and flaws. And with all this, if you give your best, it's very likely that the results you get will be quite positive.

You should also know that the seemingly difficult things that happen to you are temporary. And if you have had to experience them, it's because you have something to learn from them. Plus, you have the strength to face, cope, and overcome those things.

Ask yourself, what do I learn from this situation? That even the "hardest" situations happen for something positive in your life, even if it doesn't seem like it at the time. Everything is relative, it depends on how and where you look at the situation from.

There was a very humble family that lived in the mountains, in the Peruvian highlands. This family was made up of dad, mom and two children, and it kept growing: Mom got pregnant and brought triplets into the world. All the neighbors began to say, "Wow, how unlucky are the neighbors".

They are so poor and now they have three more children overnight". Soon after, help from the government arrived. The government said they were going to distribute free food to those who had five children or more. So that family began to receive help: food for all of them free of charge. And the neighbors began to say: "How lucky is this family".

After a while, the town governor said that those families with five or more children were going to have to leave their home and become part of a community they were building in a nearby town. They had to leave their land, their houses and in return they would be compensated with other land, other houses, and food in another town.

Neighbors began to say, "How unlucky is this family! They have to move to another community and leave their land because they are so many". A month later an avalanche destroyed the town where this family used to live. Then the neighbors began to say: "How lucky is that family! They were taken to another community and their children and their land have been saved".

As you can see, events are relative, sometimes apparently negative events that happen to you can end up being positive – they'll reveal themselves over time.

Perhaps at first you don't realize it and think that they're something negative or a misfortune. But as time goes on, it will reveal itself to you or you'll realize that this apparently negative event was finally a great blessing.

A few years ago, doctors told me I had a mediastinal tumor of four centimeters in diameter. They found it in front of the *vena cava* of my heart, behind the esophagus, between my lungs. It was impossible to do a biopsy since the area was very risky for surgery.

The nature of the tumor and the stage it was actually at when it was found, would only be seen in an open procedure (this means they needed to cut me open to have access to that specific area and be able to maneuver easily). It was my first surgery ever, so I was thought: "Wow! First time and it's such a big surgery".

My dad passed away a year before my surgery. I had moved out of the family home three months before his death. I was living alone, but after the surgery, I returned to my father's house, where my brothers and my mom took care of me.

The operation was quite big. I could not eat by myself, bathe by myself do any activity by myself. My mom was by my side day and night. One time, while she was bathing me, she told me that as a newborn, my dad, who was a doctor, was the one who bathed me and not her, because she was afraid she might drop me. I laughed and said: "Oh look, you're not off the hook anyway. Now you have to bathe me, even though I'm a grown-up" and we laughed.

I was blessed to return to my father's home thanks to that surgery. Three months later, my mom passed away. That surgery was one of the most painful surgeries I've had in my life and one of the biggest. But at the same time, I believe that surgery gave me the gift of returning home and spending more time with my mom.

I was fortunate to enjoy her presence in the last three months of her life, as we hadn't done for a long time because I was working all the time and didn't give myself enough time to be with her (although she would call me daily and we'd talk every evening). Thanks to my "bad luck" caused by the tumor, my mom and I spend time a great deal of time together.

Understand the signs life gives you... There are no coincidences.

In life, nothing happens by accident. If you look back into the past, you will realize that one situation led to another, and that last situation let once again to another. In some ways, all events are linked and correlated. Life gives you signs, like the traffic signs that tells you "go here", "go there", "stop".

You just have to pay attention and know that what happens to you is for a reason – to bring you something better. When you look at it this way and you're grateful for what happens, your attitude shifts, you start feeling more positive because you start flowing with positive energy.

How to stay calm when dealing with emotionally disturbing situations?

We've all had to face difficult situations, believe me I know… But remember that you'll never be asked for more than you can give, you will never be asked to handle situations that you can't handle. Trust your ability to deal with various situations.

Trust in yourself, in your ability to move forward with your qualities, with your flaws, with your potential, with your weaknesses, with your gifts, with who you are.

You have to know that if you've had to face a difficult situation, you have the personal resources to face them. If you don't know how, you can ask for help or ask people you trust, to give you their points of view, so you can analyze their opinion, and decide what to keep, what is useful and what isn't.

Developing your spiritual side is one of the most important things to stay calm. Relaxing and praying help increase your problem-solving skills.

I want to explain how your subconscious works, because knowing will help you put your mind in your favor. Although our mind is one, I'll divide it into two parts, just to make it easier to understand: We have the conscious part and the subconscious part.

The conscious part is the one that realizes things. It's everything that enters through your senses (what you see, hear, smell, taste or feel through touch). Everything that enters through your senses, or you realize, is conscious. The subconscious is like a fertile field, hidden in a basement. You don't know exactly what it is, but you know it exists. You don't know what is planted there, you have no idea.

What you do know is that everything that enters through your conscious part enters as orders to your subconscious, they'll be recorded after they are repeated between thirty and three hundred times.

Every day we have more than 60,000 thoughts. You see? In a few seconds, you can sow a positive or negative idea in your mind.

The subconscious has important characteristics you have to be aware of:

1. - It doesn't hear the word "No".

If I tell you "Don't think of a green elephant with a pink skirt" I bet you already saw the green elephant with a pink skirt. If I tell you "Don't think about your mother jumping rope" surely you already imagined her doing that and giggled a little. So the subconscious doesn't hear the word "no". And why doesn't it? Because the language of the mind is not the words, but the images; and the "no" doesn't have a mental representation.

The subconscious communicates through images. If I say "tree" what goes through your head? A tree appears, the T, the R, the E and the E do not appear. For this reason, when you hear "Don't think about a black dog" your mind puts the image of the black dog and that's what pops up in your head.

Remember, the "no" doesn't appear in your mind because it doesn't have a mental representation or image, so the subconscious doesn't hear it. Therefore, when you want to say something, it's preferable that you say it positively.

What does this mean? It means that you're going to say what you want without using the word "no". For example, instead of saying "I don't want to be sad", you could say "I want to be happy" or "I want to be positive". Instead of saying, "Don't forget…" you could say, "Remember…" So, say it in a positive way without using the word "no", otherwise, your mind gets the opposite message.

2. - It doesn't distinguish between true or false. It believes everything.

It believes everything you say, accepts everything, and doesn't have the capacity (unlike the conscious part), to say this is true or false. The conscious part knows this, but not the subconscious. It's like an innocent child, who believes everything. Therefore, if you say "I'm not good at writing poetry", your subconscious will believe it.

If you say "I'm so stupid!" for your subconscious it won't be something you say in the spur of the moment, it will mean "*I am stupid*", and that belief will be embedded in your mind.

Let's do an exercise that will show you in a simple way that the subconscious believes everything. Ready?

Imagine a lemon: You break the lemon and start squeezing it into your mouth. Taste the acidic lemon juice in your mouth, remember its acidic taste, as if you were eating a very acidic food or a very acid candy.

Remember that sour lemon taste in your mouth. Imagine that you place one half of the lemon on your tongue, bite down, and all the acidic juice spills into your mouth. What happened in your mouth? If you did the visualization exercise well, you may have noticed that you had a greater amount of saliva in your mouth.

Let me ask you, was the lemon real or was it imaginary? It was imaginary and yet it produced real changes in your body. Your salivary glands actually started to salivate more. You consciously knew that the lemon was imaginary, but for your subconscious it was real and it really produced real changes in your body.

3. - It tries to confirm everything that is recorded on it.

Any belief recorded into your subconscious will try to be confirmed. How? Everything you feel, say, do, how your body reacts, decisions you make, will try to confirm that your belief is true. If it's recorded in your subconscious, "Every time I eat an apple, I have the runs". Well, that's what's going to happen to you because it will try to confirm that this is true. If, for example, your subconscious recorded, "Every partner ends up leaving me". That belief will make you make decisions, attitudes, responses that make your partners leave you.

It will make sure you do things so that your partners leaves you, that is, everything you do, say, feel, how your body reacts, will confirm that partners end up leaving you, and that nobody stays with you.

4. - It pays more attention to the emotional side.

If your subconscious feels that you doubt something, it pays more attention to the emotional side. If you, for example, say: "I'm going to be calm", and suddenly you have doubts and you think, "But can I be calm?" Your subconscious will pay more attention to the emotional side, to that lingering fear, to that doubt, and you will feel uneasy.

5. - It has direct access.

The subconscious has quick and direct access to plant both positive and negative thoughts. All you have to do is enter the Alpha level.

Alpha level?

It's a consciousness state of relaxation, of tranquility, of meditation and prayer. For you to understand what Alpha level is, let me explain that the information that our senses receive is transmitted to our brain through brain cells, our neurons.

Information is transmitted through brain waves, which can go at different frequencies or cycles per second. Neurons communicate with each other through electrical impulses that we call brain waves. These waves are measured in frequency, that is, in cycles per second (the number of wavelets that pass in a second). There are four main types of brain waves:

1. - Beta waves

Beta waves involve a brain frequency of 15 to 30 cycles per second. What does this mean? It means that between 15 and 30 wavelets pass in a second. Beta brain waves appear when we are awake, like right now, while you're reading this book.

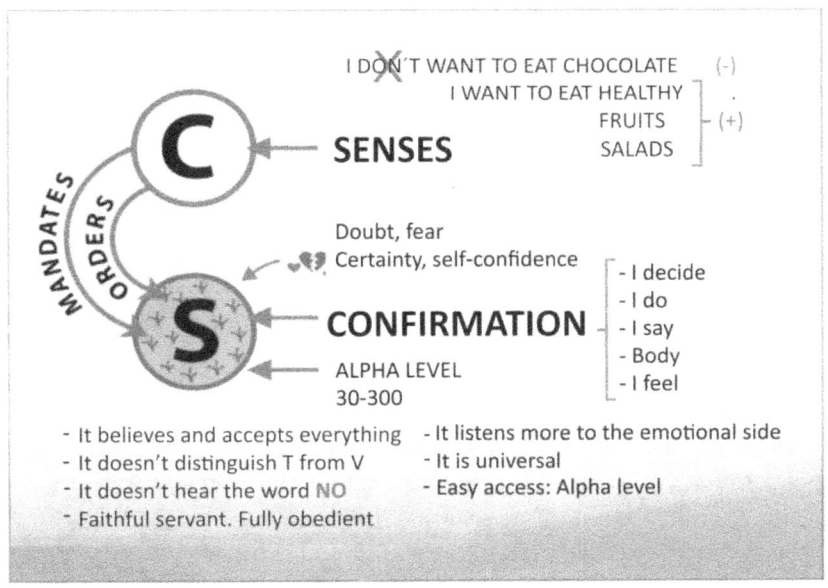

2. - Alpha waves

Alpha waves are at a frequency of 7 to 14 cycles per second. In other words, the amount of brain waves decrease per second. This is a state of relaxation, meditation, prayer, contemplation, when you're calm and at peace.

3. - Theta waves

When you're already sleepy or about to fall asleep, your brain frequency is between 4 to 7 cycles per second. This is called Theta waves.

4. - Delta waves

When you're already sleeping, your brain frequency is 4 to 0.5 cycles per second. In other words, you're already in Delta waves. Whenever you feel angry, anxious, panicky, nervous, agitated, or tense, your brain rate increases to 60 cycles per second. You're in a state of Beta consciousness, but this increased brain frequency will generate a "mental block", and alertness decreases.

A frequent example is when you're going to take a test for which you have studied, you know the answers, but you get so nervous that your mind goes "blank" and you say, "I know the answers, but I don't remember anything". This mental block is physiologically explained because of increased brain frequency.

When you're in Beta state, I could ask you, for example, "where is the room exit?" And you'll most likely point at the door. However, if in a state of relaxation at the Alpha level I could ask you, "Where is the exit?" You're going to tell me: "through the door or I could break the ceiling, break the floor or break the walls and we get out".

Problem solving increases in at the Alpha level, as well as creativity, intelligence, intuition, perception and inspiration. If an earthquake suddenly starts (your brain frequency shoots up to 60 cycles per second), and I ask you, "Where is the exit?" you'll likely feel blocked and say there is no way out because you really don't see it, even if it's in front of your eyes.

So remember that desperation won't lead you to any solution. The more nervous, anxious or tense you are, the more your mind will be blocked by the increased brain frequency that I just explained. This will prevent you from thinking of possible solutions or answers. Calm down.

The more relaxed you are, the more likely you are to find a solution. Brainstorm and ask yourself: What can I do to feel better, to feel calmer? What activities can I do to resolve the situation that concerns me and to stay calm? Everything has a solution except death.

STATE OF CONSCIOUSNESS		
15 - 30 c/s P.25	BETA	•Awake •Where is the exit?
7 - 14 c/s P.10.5	ALPHA	•Relaxation, meditation, prayer, contemplation, peace, calm. •Direct access to the subconscious • +Intelligence, creativity, perception, inspiration, intuition.
4 - 7 c/s	THETA	•Sleepy
4 - 0.5 c/s	DELTA	•Sleepy •Sleep
60 c/s	BETA	•Anger, anxiety, panic, scared, tense, agitated, nervous •"Mental blockage", reduced lucidity.

What can help you significantly is to face situations one by one, step by step. Divide that problematic huge monster situation into small situations, into smaller parts to face them and move forward in their solution. What often paralyzes you is how you see the situation, not the situation itself.

You see the problem as a boogeyman that is "too big" to deal with. However, scientific studies reveal that when facing a difficult situation, reality isn't even 10% of what you feared so much.

Imagine that you see the shadow of a monster on the wall, and you think: "How am I going to be able to face this?" But as you get closer, you see it's only a little mouse, but its shadow on the wall reflected the image of a monster. Your mind will probably make the problem look bigger (about 90% more than it really is). However, by the time you decide to tackle the situation, it will be much easier than you had imagined (only 10% of what you thought it was).

What paralyzes you is the assumption: the image you created in your mind. But not because it looks like that in your mind, it means it's true. Therefore, it's important you take the first steps to face the situation, instead of rushing, avoiding or postponing it.

And when you face the "difficult" situation, you will realize that it wasn't as terrible as you thought. Step by step, with baby steps, you'll find solutions to your problems.

If you realize you need help, as someone with experience on the field, I can tell you, I can say you're just a phone call away. Learn to ask for help, no matter how intelligent and capable you are. You won't necessarily have the solution to all your problems. Everyone has different knowledge in different areas, some more, others less and it's OK.

You can ask the opinion of someone with more experience or knowledge than you in the area you need help with. Later on, you can draw your own conclusions and decide what to do.

Remember that there is no single way to solve problems. There are multiple ways to solve them. Even if your financial situation is affecting you, you should know that you can't only get money by doing what you did all your life. You can be creative and see how you can reinvent yourself. You can do other types of activities that can also generate income.

For example, Joaquín and Pablo worked as accountants, but due to a crisis in the company they worked at, they were fired. They liked music, they started to get together to create songs, to record video clips and they reinvented themselves. Their current job is music production.

You probably know some other examples of people who reinvented themselves in order to generate some extra money through activities they liked. Remember, there are several ways to do it. Water doesn't come from a single source. You have to keep walking with hope, exploring, searching like a child, experimenting at peace and enjoying the journey.

Pay attention to the signs life brings. When you least expect it, you'll have found that special thing that you're looking for, and that will cross your path when you least expect it.

How can you feel happy in situations that throw your heart into turmoil?

You are able to face what's happening to you. Even when you feel you can't do it, you need to trust your personal and spiritual resources, and that you'll be able to move forward. Also trust that you have God's help or the help of the higher beings you believe in. When your mind is in positive state, you begin to attract those positive situations you visualized.

If you want to achieve positive results even in difficult situations, start sowing what you want in your subconscious, feeling as if you have already accomplished it - Remember, your subconscious believes everything!

Another important point: everything is temporary. What is happening to you is going to pass, it's something temporary. You have enough personal resources to face it and overcome the situation. If you look closely, you will realize that many of the difficult situations you experience are bringing out the best of your personal resources. Believe that they are like hard workouts, and that after every one of them, you'll be stronger.

Every difficult situation is training a part of you, it's helping you improve that part of you that you'll have to use to overcome the situation. When it's over (because it's temporary and it will pass), you'll feel more secure and more self-confident.

Be happy because you're improving as a human being. After all, you'll discover that you have personal resources you had no idea you had. The feeling of personal satisfaction will be amazing. Will you dare to rediscover yourself through seemingly difficult situations?

How to keep a good attitude towards life?

It's important to know that every situation happens for something positive in your life. It's about discovering what gift the situation brings. Maybe this gift came to you in a damaged, dirty box; but, inside it hold a special gift for you. You have to learn how to look beyond.

The difficult situation is only the tip of the iceberg, it's what you see at first. What you have to learn to look at is deep down, and as yourself what gift is this difficult or apparently difficult situation bringing me? What part of me needs to be trained with this challenge? What personal capacity will I discover through this difficult situation I'm facing today?

God or life won't put you in situations you can't handle. The difficult situation comes to you with the hidden solution. First you need to calm down and look patiently and carefully where the solution is. Every problem has a hidden solution. Your job is to unravel the puzzle, find the solution that is right there.

You just have to look at the situation calmly, so that you can uncover one of the solutions.

Another element that will help you keep a good attitude is a high positive personal vibration. But how can you do it? One of the ways is to be thankful for what's positive in your life. Most people tend to focus only on the problem. But this is about appreciating your life in a broad way, recognizing that not everything in your life is problems, that there are areas of your life that are very healthy, beautiful, for which you feel grateful.

Yes, grateful because you can walk, you can breathe, you can see, you can feed yourself, because something or someone special exists. So, being thankful is one of the ways to stay positive because it generates a good vibration to recognize the good that life gives you.

If there is a black dot on a white board, you don't need to always complain about it. On the contrary, you can be grateful you have a white board, realizing that the largest percentage of the white board is clean. A dot is just a dot on the board. Don't let that black dot cloud your vision and make you forget that you have a whole white board.

Another way to increase your personal vibration is by sharing what you know, what you have and mainly what you are. Sharing yourself, giving yourself (not just sharing or giving), exponentially increases your personal vibration. Giving part of your time, part of your life. When you have a gift or a skill, you have to share it.

When I was little, whenever I read or listened to the parable of the talents from the Bible (Matthew 25: 14-30), to be honest I didn't much and I asked myself, "Why is it that whoever has more is given more and to who has barely anything, even that is taken away?"

Let me share the parable of the talents with you: Listen to this too. A man going on a journey, called his servants and entrusted his wealth to them. To one he gave five bags of gold, to another two bags, and to another one bag, each according to his ability. Then he went on his journey. The man who had received five bags of gold went at once and put his money to work and gained five bags more. So also, the one with two bags of gold gained two more. But the man who had received one bag went off, dug a hole in the ground and hid his master's money.

After a long time the master of those servants returned and settled accounts with them. The man who had received five bags of gold brought the other five. "Master", he said, "you entrusted me with five bags of gold. See, I have gained five more". His master replied, "Well done, good and faithful servant! You have been faithful with a few things; I will put you in charge of many things.

Come and share your master's happiness!"

The man with two bags of gold also came. "Master", he said, "you entrusted me with two bags of gold; see, I have gained two more". His master replied, "Well done, good and faithful servant! You have been faithful with a few things; I will put you in charge of many things.

Come and share your master's happiness!" Then the man who had received one bag of gold came. "Master" he said "I knew that you are a hard man, harvesting where you have not sown and gathering where you have not scattered seed. So I was afraid and went out and hid your gold in the ground. See, here is what belongs to you".

His master replied "You wicked, lazy servant! So you knew that I harvest where I have not sown and gather where I have not scattered seed?" Well, then, you should have put my money on deposit with the bankers, so that when I returned I would have received it back with interest. "So take the bag of gold from him and give it to the one who has ten bags".

For whoever has will be given more, and they will have an abundance. Whoever does not have, even what they have will be taken from them. And throw that worthless servant outside, into the darkness, where there will be weeping and gnashing of teeth".

I have to refer to the fact that a gold talent is equivalent to an approximate measure of 34 kg of gold. Can you imagine how much money that represents today? Nowadays, one talent of gold would be worth approximately US $ 385,380. Did you notice the difference between the attitude of those two servants who received five and two talents respectively, and the servant who received one talent?

The first two knew that whoever gave them those talents trusted them and was also self-confident. They trusted in their abilities and invested their time and qualities to multiply what they were given.

In your case, if you want to improve in any aspect or area of your life (your trade or profession, your interpersonal relationships, your ability to do crafts, your sports), it's important that you dedicate enough time to grow in that aspect and get the best results. On the other hand, we see that the servant who received only one talent probably felt afraid or lazy to work on it or wasn't really interested.

Have you ever wondered if your attitude of fear, disinterest or laziness is what may be stopping you and causing you to lose your stability and even what you have now? Carefully observe how fear paralyzes you. Fear of risking, of failing and laziness can also paralyze you. Fear and laziness keep you in your comfort zone, a comfortable situation that is familiar to you. A situation you don't necessarily like, but that you learned to deal with.

For example, you prefer to watch television and say that the money is not enough, thank making the effort and invest time in doing something different, a new business or project. Do you see how fear or laziness means that we could love even that one talent we have?

As a child I didn't understand this parable very well, but then I realized that these talents represented the abilities that God gives us all! I learned that when we put our skills into practice, they grow, they multiply, and if we share them and teach them to others, they will multiply even more, because we could awaken new abilities in these people or they could discover their own abilities.

On the other hand, the person who has abilities, but doesn't use them, that is, doesn't take action, loses it until those abilities eventually disappear. I understood that this parable was a call precisely to use the abilities, the gifts that God has given each one of us. He has given each of us even one gift. We don't need twenty skills, one is enough.

If we put it into practice, we enhance it, and we'll probably discover that we have new skills, that they will multiply, grow, and if we share them with others, we will create a positive chain that keeps on giving.

What helps you stay positive?

There are three main aspects that can help you stay positive:

1. - Personal resources or things you can do to keep your own positive attitude.

2. - Family and friends, the people you love and love you – your pet too!

3. - Having God or a deep spiritual life. It is very important.

Something that helps a lot on a personal level is trusting yourself, trusting that life will bring you unexpected gifts, trusting that God is on your side, and that all those things or situations that happen in your life are for or for something positive.

Another thing that helps a lot is to wake up and thank God for life, being able to wake up every day, for being healthy, for giving you the gift of having your family and even for the presence of your pet that plays with you and gives you lots of affection.

Be grateful for the parents you have or had, be grateful that God guides you every day. Be certain that He will place the clues along your path to lead you towards your goals and your dreams.

It also helps you to keep a positive attitude if you do activities that you like, projects, plans, hobbies, things that you don't "have" to do, but you do it just to enjoy yourself.

It helps a lot when you find God through the people you're blessed to deal with each day.

Through them, the Lord continues to teach you and continues to give you his friendship and love.

Knowing that there are people out there with a positive, hopeful outlook on life, despite the difficult situations they may go through, helps you look at life with optimism.

It also helps to relax, do different fun activities, get out of the routine, have even small moments to do simple activities such as going around the park, riding a bike, playing for a while with your pet, writing a poem, painting, drawing, making a stamp, watering the garden. Small different activities will fill your day to day with color.

Frequent physical activity for thirty or forty minutes (without stopping) generates endorphins, which are natural antidepressants. In addition to improving your mood, it will decrease your stress and you will feel calmer.

What physical activities can you do? You have thousands to choose from: walking, running, dancing, exercising, sweeping, mopping, cleaning windows, jumping rope, playing tag, taking your puppy for a walk, swimming, surfing, etc.

Turn "I can't" into "How can I?"

I remember that an old plumber would come to my house, that every time he encountered a problem and did not know exactly how to solve it, instead of saying "I can't solve it", he immediately said, "How can I solve this?" Within seconds, he came up with ways how he could solve the situation.

The interesting thing here is that he was using what we know as pre-assumptions. He assumed he was going to be able to solve the problem. He spoke in a positive way (How can I?). Right there, he was saying that he could. The idea is to find out the way, the how.

Whenever you ask your mind "How can I do this?" it will answer you back. So if you simply ask your question with the included affirmation that your mind can do it, it will quickly give you an answer. The type of response you get is really just a reflection of the quality of the questions you ask yourself. The simpler the question, the more options and answers you'll get.

If you complicate the question or make it sound "too big", you will block your mind and the answers will take longer to come.

For example, if you ask yourself: "What business can I do right now to make a million dollars a month?" Your mind is probably going to feel a bit intimidated and it will take a moment or a long time to respond.

But if you ask yourself: "What small steps could I take to make a dollar a day?" You'll most likely get lots of answers. When this "small" brainstorming comes out (yes, in quotation marks), you can then combine them and create something very interesting with great results.

Do you know what I do when I don't know how to solve something? I immediately ask God for help, I say: "Help me, please show me what to do. I want to be a good channel, let me be a good instrument, but please help me so everything goes well".

Connecting with nature also helps you keep a positive attitude (the greenness, the fields, the flowers, the sky with its nights, its sunsets and sunrises, the sea, the breeze, the river, etc.), listening to instrumental music (it relaxes you, calms you down and improves the flow of ideas), giving and receiving hugs (when the COVID-19 pandemic ends, to be safe).

Let me share with you that what helps me most to keep a positive attitude in life is my relationship with God.

It helps me to ray, thank, entrust each of my projects in God's hands, and offer Him all my work, my day to day, my life also. I also know I have our mother from heaven, Mary, who is always interceding for us and loves us (I respect those who have different beliefs).

And the most beautiful thing of all is to realize that the Lord knows what I'm made of. He loves me and accepts me as I am and that even with all my limitations, He counts on me to help others.

God knows what you're made of, and even with the limitations you may have, He loves you, accepts you and leads you along those paths where you can feel at peace and happy with yourself and add positively to the lives of people who are fortunate to meet you.

Thoughts that help keep a good attitude.
If one door closes, three doors open.
Everything I give, comes back multiplied. Everything happens for something positive, always.
God is always on my side, even if sometimes it doesn't seem like it. Life is beautiful, despite everything.
Friends are angels who lend us their wings, when we forget how to fly.
Thank you, thank you and thank you.
Always move forward!
If I had to live or go through this, it's because I can do it, otherwise, it wouldn't have happened.
God puts the most difficult tests on his best warriors. Do you want to have excuses or do you want to have results?
One more step...
When you don't know how to do something, ask God for help. Any situation, no matter how difficult it may seem, has a solution. Everything has a solution, except death.

You need to have everything under control.
Have you ever felt that when you're not in control of things, you feel anxious and in order to be calm, for example, at work, you need to be aware of what is happening in each area or know what each colleague in the team is working?
The need to be in control becomes obvious. This can happen to you in different areas of your life (home, school, work, friendships, various activities).
When you realize that you're not in control of things at certain times and situations, intense restlessness, anxiety and irritability generally come into play.
What do you need to do to handle this need to get things under control? Trust your responsiveness. Look at the evidence, you'll realize that in various situations you have faced, even when you did not have all the variables under control, you were able to respond adequately and obtained very good results.
What's important is that you know what the goal is or what objective you're aiming for and trust that when the variables you need come along, you'll have the ability to work with them and combine them in such a way that they give you the expected result.

It's like you want to cook a stew and suddenly you don't see the meat, the potatoes, the salt, the onion, the oil (each ingredient is somewhere in the kitchen). You don't need to have all the condiments and items in sight to start cooking. You have to trust that the moment you have all the ingredients on the table you will have the ability to combine them properly, you will know what to do with each ingredient and you'll obtain an excellent result.

Can you imagine what it would be like if we psychiatrists, psychologists, psychotherapists, coaches, needed to have everything under control? What would it be like if we needed to know what each client or each patient is going to talk about in each session? As you can imagine, each session with each person is unique, and each one brings his or her own subject.

We're not fortune tellers and we don't know what topic they will bring to each session. So we have to trust our responsiveness. We have to trust our knowledge and experience and that our approach can help them adequately.

Since the beginning of my career, what helped me a great deal to have confidence in myself and that I was going to be able to help my patients, regardless of the case, was that I prayed to God and asked him: "Please send me to the patients that You know that I will be able to help, those who are not, please send them to another doctor who can help them".

And, sure, it may sound funny, but this sentence really helped me a lot because when a patient came to my office for help, I worked with the conviction that I would be able to help them, because I had already asked God for this. Therefore, I said to myself, "if the patient is already here with me, it's because I'll be able to help him/her, and I worked (and keep working) with this confidence and certainty.

Another thing that helps a lot is to trust the experience, the life lessons, your knowledge. Look at the evidence. Remember situations in which you didn't have things under control, i.e., you did not know how everything was going in every single detail, and yet, when you had to show results, you did well.

Keyla didn't believe in her ability to respond to unexpected events and she felt the "need" to have everything under control. I told her: "You work in personal training, right? What happens if one day in the middle of the session, your client injures his/her arm and you had just planned to do an arm exercise routine in that session?

Imagine your client asks you to continue with other types of exercises that exclude arms. Are you going to cancel the training session because you hadn't prepared other alternative routines?"

Obviously not, you'll check your personal internal resources, and you'll suggest other exercise routines. You have those personal resources (experience, knowledge) you can turn to whenever you need them, you have to trust that you know your subject and that you have that responsiveness".

When you have to face unexpected situations where certain answers don't depend on you, believe that you will solve them well. If it hadn't been like that, I don't think you would be here until now; you would have stayed halfway on the path. Remember that not all results will be perfect. Perfect is an enemy of good. When something cannot be done in a certain way, there will always be a thousand and more alternatives to do it, in different ways.

Approaching different situations from different angles, from different perspectives, listening to different voices allows you to expand your capacity to react and respond appropriately to each situation and diversify options. Being open to having that spontaneous response has to do with being sure that there is an immense range of reaction possibilities, within you, in each situation.

There is no single solution. There could be many, with different tones and shades, all of them with beautiful results. You have to trust that all that palette of colors, of response nuances you have within yourself whenever it is necessary. They will come out in the best way, regardless of the situation you are in.

If you're certain that all the colors of nature are in you, you'll remain calm and peaceful. You won't need to look at all the colors to feel that you're in control of the situation or to trust your good results. Many times the unexpected generates incredible, beautiful nuances that will surprise you. It is beautiful and interesting when you allow yourself to be positively surprised by life and by yourself, with your answer. Give yourself the opportunity to enjoy that spontaneous and colorful response in you.

Trust that whenever you need give an answer, solve something, even if you don't have all the elements in sight or things under control, you'll bring out what is in you and come up a work of art. Trust yourself.

Thanks? For what?

To be grateful is to simultaneously generate and send positive energy to whoever had a nice gesture with you. When you give thanks, you're learning to receive, to recognize the good that has come into your life, be it through an attitude, something material or a situation. When you recognize and appreciate the good or sometimes the difficult situation you have to face, somehow that positive vibration will attract more positive circumstances into your life. Remember to always be grateful.

How to face challenges without fear?

Challenges, new, different or difficult situations generate concern, uncertainty, doubts and even fear in all of us. If you wait for the fear to disappear before taking action, you will never do anything. The idea is to do, despite the fear, and it will fade away as you keep going. Little by little, that restlessness will calm down and when you begin to realize that you're able to take small steps, to move forward, your self-confidence and your efficacy will increase. Brave is not the one who is not afraid, but the one who faces fear the longest.

Believing in God and developing a spiritual life will help you have strength and confidence to face different difficult situations. Knowing that you're not alone is knowing that you belong to a great family, that we are all one, and that we all walk with the desire that each one of us who make up this world is happy and can take care of our world, together.

It's very important to learn to share and work as a team, appreciating each other as the human beings we are, without discriminating, accepting ourselves as we are, respecting our diversity and racial, socioeconomic, religious, sexual choice differences, learning to walk together, and helping each other towards common goals.

When I was a medical student, they asked for volunteers for a vaccination day for the population. I signed up and they divided us in teams. Each team included a doctor, a nurse, a nursing technician and a dentist, that is, four people. The team consisted of an evangelical girl, another Jehovah's Witness girl, the boy was an atheist and I was a Catholic.

In the area where we had to go give the shots, we had to climb a hill, the little houses were located in almost extreme spots, and the winding roads were made of dirt and stone. The vaccines were in a cooler. One alone could not climb the hill with that cooler because the hill was very steep.

What we did to raise the box was to stand one after the other, we handed it along, from the bottom up. We worked as a human ladder, with the only goal of reaching the last house on the hill to vaccinate the kids who lived there.

When all this happened, I realized that the four of us, even with different religious beliefs, had come together and helped each other to climb that hill and finally reach our common goal, which was to vaccinate the last child in the last little house on the top of the hill. This made me think and realize that it didn't matter if we had different beliefs (in this case religious) but that the four of us had the same goal: to vaccinate all the children assigned to us.

Although the job included reaching little house at the top of that mountain, we felt so rewarded to realize that in the end what was important wasn't our differences, but our common goal. We focused more on what united us, on the positive goal we wanted to achieve for the well-being and protection to our population.

When we want to achieve a goal and we have to ask for help or we have to share work with other people, we can look at ourselves as human beings, who go together towards a goal, without stopping or being distracted by our differences. I was wondering if we allow this to become an obstacle or focus on the common goal. Do we become human bridges to move forward together towards the same goal?

When the four of us introduced ourselves, we smiled to discover that we each had different religious beliefs. However, the whole day was very pleasant. We walked together, we climbed that mountain together, we helped each other. There were even times when one could not go up and we all held hands to help the other climb, and we really became a human ladder. This was an unforgettable and beautiful experience because, as I said, our common goal mattered more than our different religious beliefs.

What does it mean to live fully here and now?

It's important that you're connected to your present without looking back to the past or creating images of the future. Live day by day. Be present with your five senses in each situation and in each moment you have to face. Be connected to what you have to live today, what already happened is in the past and you can't change it.

Regarding the future, you really don't know what's going to happen. Many things can change from here on. New resources can be created. There can be different solutions. Worrying is not worth it, it's better to focus on the present moment (when it happens). It's also important to be connected with the signs that life gives you. Many times life sends you unexpected gifts and you need to be attentive to those little details to feel the blessing that God or life gives you every day.

A few years ago, I visited the Peruvian jungle. I remember a long walk in the middle of the thick vegetation. We had to climb some winding paths. We had walked so much that I was honestly exhausted and started using a wooden stick to keep walking. The group was already ahead, and we were going towards a waterfall. I walked and stopped for short breaks, and after a while I didn't see the group anymore.

I was walking alone, and suddenly I turn around and see a blue butterfly flying by my side, so I said, "Wow. What a beautiful butterfly!" and I continued walking slowly. Then I realized that when I stopped, the butterfly would stop flying at the same place where I stopped, even if I stopped for just ten or twenty seconds.

I kept moving forward and the butterfly kept moving next to me and I said, "Oh it must be a coincidence". However, I stopped again and the butterfly also stopped at the same stop. I kept moving forward and the butterfly kept moving forward too.

I stopped again and the butterfly stopped again, and so I was entertained, watching if the butterfly flew at the same pace as my walking for more than fifteen minutes, and finally when I was able to see the group already near the waterfall, the butterfly took off and left me there. For me, her company was a blessing – it was a gift from God and from life. I was so fascinated with the butterfly that I forgot I was so tired and was able to keep walking, I was able to get to the edge of the waterfall and find my group.

Those are the gifts that God and life give us. If we pay attention, we will enjoy them, we will be deeply grateful and that will fill us with energy and positive vibration. This will help us keep a positive attitude in the face of difficult situations. Along the way, we will find those "oases" where we can drink fresh water, rest and take a break from the intense heat.

How can you find what makes you happy?

Listening to yourself and watching yourself. See what activity makes your time fly by, what you enjoy, what makes you smile, what is it that you talk about the most or what you like to talk about. Explore around because it's not just one thing, situation or person that is going to make you happy. Being happy has to do with finding makes you really happy from within.

Sharing can also make you happy. Learning to receive is as important as learning to give, because when you learn to receive you allow the person who gives you to also feel the joy of being able to share something.

Imagine that you want to give a ball to a child, you do it with the best intention and he says, "No thanks, I don't want any gift from you"; On the other hand, if that child receives the ball and says "Thank you" and you see him playing happily, how you feel?

Always remember that giving is as important as receiving.

One night I had gone to get some take-out, but before I got home I stopped at a gas station to get some gas. A little boy came up to me. He was about seven years old and was selling some gum. The boy told me, "Miss, two chewing gums for one *sol*". The chewing gums sold on the streets were five for one *sol*. I hadn't even seen what gum the boy was selling, but I told him "At least give me three chewing gums for one *sol*" and he said, "OK, miss".

When he handed me the three pieces of gum for one *sol*, I realized that it was a chewing gum that cost much more than what I was paying. The price that the boy had asked me for two chewing gums for one *sol* was only fair. Despite that, he was handing me three pieces of gum. At that moment I was moved, because I said, "Despite his poverty, this child is giving me a little more for this price, he gives more than what he can afford". So I took all the food I was bringing home and asked him: "Are you hungry? Have you eaten anything?" I handed him the food, but told him I had no utensils.

He said "Don't worry", he took out the lid of a soda bottle and began to eat. He sat down on the floor and called his friends who came over when they saw he had some food.

I received from that child more than he could really afford to give, but he wanted to give it away and so he did. That made me want to give him even more. There, by doing that I truly understood what "give and you shall receive" meant.

When you give and give yourself, you generate a positive attitude in other people, that good desire, those good vibrations. And then life, others or yourself will give you back that positive energy, that positive vibration that will help you have the ability to positively face those situations that "torment" your life (whatever they may be).

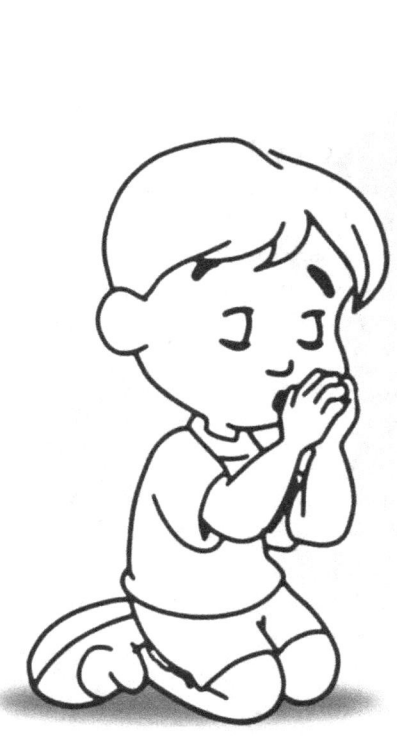

EPILOGUE

Dear friend,

Thank you for giving me the opportunity to walk by your side. I loved sharing my experiences with you. From the bottom of my heart, I hope I have given you a new outlook (hopefully a more positive one) for those situations that "torment" your life and that from now on you can look at things from different perspectives to make your journey a bit lighter.

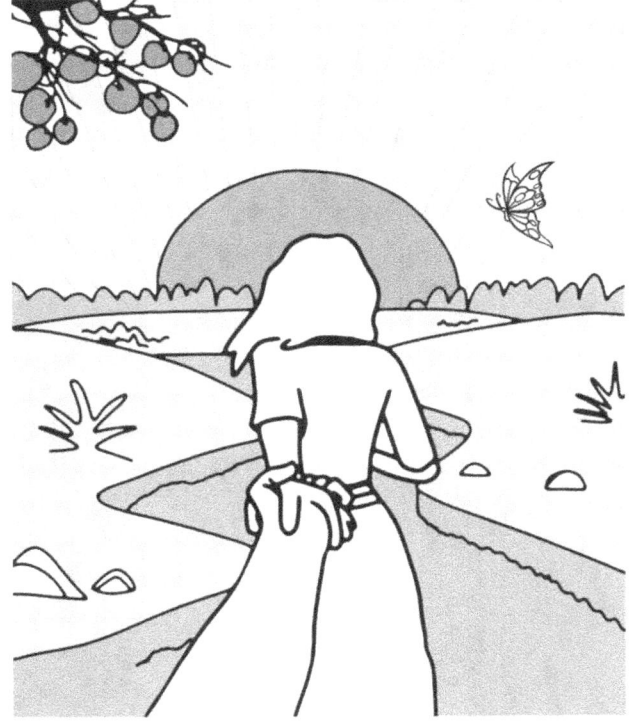

Until we meet again!

Susana Yoshiyama Miyagusuku.

www.ingramcontent.com/pod-product-compliance
Lightning Source LLC
Chambersburg PA
CBHW032211220526
45472CB00018B/1100